AN ESSENTIAL BOOK FOR EVERY PARENT
EAR INFECTIONS IN YOUR CHILD

"Clear...easy to read...a must for anyone whose child has recurrent ear infections." **—*Washington Parent***

"A comprehensive source of information."
—National Association for Hearing and Speech Action

"This excellent work presents a clear and comprehensive layman's guide to understanding this chronic children's malady....Highly recommended." **—*Booklist***

"A clear and comprehensive guide to a problem that confronts numerous children and their parents."
—Carol Krucoff, Health Editor, *Washington Post*

"Required reading for parents of the 'otitis prone' child....Dr. Grundfast and Ms. Carney tell what is known about children's ear disease in a way that is both complete and approachable."
—Glenn Isaacson, M.D., Department of Pediatric Otolaryngology, Children's Hospital of Pittsburgh

"A great service to the public."
—Erdem I. Cantekin, Ph.D., Professor of Otolaryngology, University of Pittsburgh School of Medicine

(continued on next page)

KENNETH GRUNDFAST, M.D., is Chairman of the Department of Otolaryngology of Children's Hospital National Medical Center in Washington, D.C.

CYNTHIA J. CARNEY is a health writer and a former contributor to the *Washington Post* health section. Her articles have also appeared in *Commonweal* and *Ms*.

EAR INFECTIONS
IN YOUR CHILD

Kenneth Grundfast, M.D.
and
Cynthia J. Carney

Illustrations by Joyce Hurwitz

WARNER BOOKS

A Warner Communications Company

Warner Books Edition
Copyright © 1987 by Kenneth Grundfast and Cynthia J. Carney
All rights reserved.
This Warner Books edition is published by arrangement with Compact Books,
2131 Hollywood Boulevard, Hollywood, Florida 33020

Warner Books, Inc., 666 Fifth Avenue, New York, NY 10103

Ⓦ A Warner Communications Company

Printed in the United States of America
First Warner Books Printing: July 1989
10 9 8 7 6 5 4 3 2 1

Library of Congress Cataloging-in-Publication Data

Grundfast, Kenneth.
    Ear Infections in your child.

    Otitis media in children — popular works.
I. Carney, Cynthia J.   II. Title. [DNLM: 1. Otitis —
in infancy & childhood — popular works. WV   200   G889e]
RF225.G783   618.92′098′4   87-7538
ISBN 0-446-38931-5 (pbk.) (U.S.A.)
ISBN 0-446-38932-3 (pbk.) (Can.)

Acknowledgments

B ecause so many different fields of medicine touch upon the treatment of otitis media, the authors interviewed many specialists—from anesthesiologists to speech therapists. We thank all the people who answered our many questions and helped us so enthusiastically gather information for our book. We would like especially to thank: Gilbert Herer, Ph.D., Chairman, and the staff, of the Hearing and Speech Department at Children's Hospital National Medical Center in Washington, D.C.; Richard Schwartz, M.D., pediatrician and researcher in Vienna, Va.; Marion P. Downs, MA, DHS, professor emitera, Department of Otolaryngology, University of Colorado Health Sciences Center; the staff of the Department of Otolaryngology at Children's Hospital National Medical Center—Sue Heidig, R.N., Mary Jo Palmer, Debra Knight, Gregory Milmoe, M.D.; Deborah Gilbert, Director of Medical Library at Children's Hospital National Medical Center; Cheryl Levitt, R.N.; Iona Razi, M.D.; Lee Ann Slayton, public education coordinator for the Association for Care of Children's Health; and the many parents who told us their personal stories and volunteered their children to be used as "models" for photographs in our book. A special thanks to Notoco Inc. for contributing toward the cost of photographs.

Finally, we'd like to thank our families for supporting us through many months of deadlines and late nights at the computer and on the telephone: Gregory Byrne and Brendan Carney Byrne; Cay and Bob Byrne; Hildie Carney; Ruthanne, Rena and Dara Grundfast.

Contents

ix

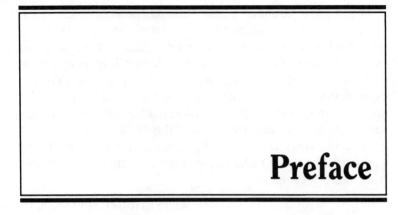

Preface

FROM A DOCTOR'S POINT OF VIEW

As I have taken care of children with ear infections during the past several years, I have come to realize that many parents want to know more about the causes and treatment of their children's ear infections. I have had the feeling that parents could understand and absorb more information than ordinarily is provided by doctors. The impetus for parents seeking additional information seems to be that parents want to be sure they are doing the right thing for their children when they give medication or consent to a surgical procedure. The more information parents have, the more secure they feel in making decisions about care for their children.

In writing this book, my goal has been one of providing relevant information in a concise and easily readable format. Hopefully, the information has been presented in a way that is understandable yet not overly simplified. After all, though all parents have many questions about childhood ear infections, sometimes there are not direct and straightforward answers. Doctors themselves do not yet have all the answers about causes and treatment of ear infections.

If you are a parent of a child who has been troubled by ear infections and you want to play a more active role in the management of your child's ear infections, I hope that this book will enable you to achieve an understanding of a problem that has seemed frustrating and bewildering to you. Then, I hope that you will gain the confidence to consider yourself a well informed participant in decisionmaking rather than a helpless bystander. If only parents find this book helpful in terms of allaying fears and clarifying misconceptions, then I will know that the hours that went into research and writing of this book were well spent.

—KENNETH GRUNDFAST, M.D.

FROM A PARENT'S POINT OF VIEW ▬▬

It was to be a routine office visit to check my ten-month-old son's ears two weeks after an acute ear infection. But it turned into a nightmare for me—one that I'll never forget. The ENT specialist suddenly announced that he was going to perform a myringotomy (lancing of the eardrum). And before I could even open my mouth to ask what a myringotomy was, the nurse had already entered the room and was getting together the instruments, and an assistant had already started wrapping in a papoose my frightened and howling son. Panic gripped me and clouded my mind—and within minutes my son was handed to me and I whisked him out the door. At home, after I comforted my son and calmed myself down, I resolved never to allow emotions to lock my tongue and cloud my mind through the intimidation of a physician.

That incident occurred only two months after my son Brendan's first ear infection. It was a turning point, however, in how I would approach Brendan's medical care throughout the years he suffered recurrent ear infections. I decided to seek answers about ear infections on my own because I wasn't getting answers from my physicians. And when I found very little information about childhood ear infections in childcare manuals, Dr. Grundfast and I decided it was time to fill the gap in an area that affects so many children and so many parents' pocketbooks.

Many other scenes are etched in my memory regarding Brendan's illnesses: the time my heart stopped when a pediatrician looked in my son's ears, furrowed her brow as she looked at me and said, "He's got such a bad ear infection. It's just full of pus." Or the time I blindly accepted a pediatrician's earnest assurances that parents should not bother learning how to examine their child's ears at home. Or the endless 30 minutes that my husband and I sat in the hospital's waiting room while my eleven-month-old son was having tubes put into his ears. The scenes combine with a blur of sleepless nights, visits to doctors, struggles with administering antibiotics and days of holding and comforting my lethargic and feverish child.

At least two positive developments have come from these bad times: first, I have taken a much more active role in the health care of my family by questioning all medication and procedures until I fully understand the rationale and consequences of the treatment. Second, this book has been written, and it is my hope it will help ease the anxiety of other parents in my situation.

Now that I have co-authored a book about childhood ear infections, do I have all the answers to my son's illness? Unfortunately, no. Even as I was researching and writing, I had to cancel many appointments and shut off my word processor many times to nurse Brendan back to health from an ear infection. Neither myself nor my physicians understand why Brendan has had continual ear infections since he was eight months old, and my husband and I have finally accepted that we will never know the reasons.

What my husband and I have learned, however, is that it's very harmful—and a waste of valuable energy—for parents to agonize and blame themselves for an illness they can't control. Our mental anguish was probably far greater than the physical pain or discomfort experienced by our son. And, although babies seem fragile and vulnerable to painful ear infections, they are able to recover quickly with good care and—in the vast majority of cases—carry on with their busy lives as if nothing ever happened.

What will I do differently if I have another child who suffers recurrent ear infections? First, I will have a more realistic perspective on the illness, realizing that ear infections are not life threatening if treated properly. I also will bear in mind that ear infections are a normal part of childhood illness, although some children have more infections than others. Second, I will ask my doctor more questions, no matter how "dumb" they may seem (and I won't apologize for asking them). Third, I'll limit my child's medication to times when he is severely ill. Finally, I'll be more content in knowing that I'm not the only parent who's going through this struggle—and that there's now a book that can answer the questions I once wanted to ask.

CYNTHIA J. CARNEY

Introduction

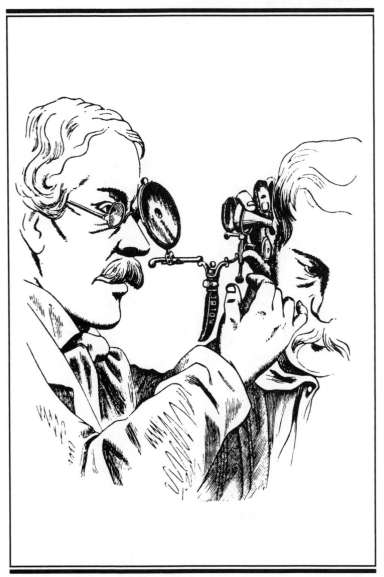

"Weber's Reflector." Illustration from *Diseases of the Ear*. Laurence Turnbull, M.D. JP Lippincott & Co. 1872.

Introduction

Ear infection. Mention those words to a group of parents and you're likely to hear a panorama of first-hand stories, complaints and fears. Some parents will say they're concerned about the all-too-frequent presence of antibiotics in their home. Others are losing faith in a once-trusted pediatrician who is unable to curb relentless ear infections. Yet another parent questions the need for the insertion of ear tubes.

These parents are afraid. Many of them often consider the hidden middle ear system as a delicate, mysterious and temperamental mechanism. They erroneously fear that something terrible—deafness? brain disease?—will happen if the ear infection isn't treated properly and immediately, or if one dose of medicine is missed.

These parents are frustrated. Ear infections continue to plague their children despite the best efforts of the medical profession and costly medical bills.

These parents are confused. One doctor prescribes a course of antibiotics over several months, another adopts a "wait-and-see" approach, and another immediately refers the child

3

to an ear specialist for insertion of tubes. These physicians' recommendations may seem random, inconsistent and arbitrary.

The initial fear, anxiety, guilt and confusion can soon lead to anger, frustration and skepticism once a child's condition becomes chronic. To many parents, the specter of otitis media is hovering over their family at all times. At a time when doctors can transplant organs, sustain life in premature babies and rebuild limbs, parents are confounded by the lack of a magical cure for ear infections, and their feeling of helplessness grows.

What's a Parent to Do?

But there *is* something positive parents can do to help a child suffering from recurrent ear infections. They can begin to seek an active role in finding proper medical care. That means parents must start reading, asking more questions of doctors and being more observant of their children. This active approach to participating in medical care is an idea that is becoming more accepted in our consumer-oriented and health-conscious society as specialized magazines, self-help books and television programs bring the world of medicine into the American home.

Who has the right answers about childhood ear infections? Your pediatrician? Your friend's pediatrician? The latest article in a parents' magazine? Trying to sift through the mound of often-conflicting information is enough to make parents throw their hands up in despair.

What Can You Expect From This Book?

Ear Infections In Your Child is a comprehensive source for parents on otitis media. It is not a textbook, although much of the information is derived from textbooks on anatomy, microbiology and pediatric otolaryngology (the study of the ear, nose and throat in children). It discusses the causes, treatment and prevention of ear infections and gives a few basics about medical science in order to explain middle ear function.

However, the book is intended to reach far beyond the basics of childhood ear infections. The authors identify and explore the social and economic forces contributing to the increase in ear infections in the U.S., discuss ways you can establish a working relationship with your physician, and discuss the ongoing controversies among experts in otitis media.

Since every physician approaches treatment of chronic ear infections differently, this book will not please every doctor all of the time. For every piece of advice offered in the following pages, at least one physician would advise differently. The authors hope that small quibbles over bits of advice in this book do not interfere with its goal: to provide a source of information for parents to be used in conjunction with advice received from a physician. The authors believe that even a simple accomplishment such as beginning a dialogue between parent and physician is justification for the long hours spent researching and writing this book.

How to Use This Book

Ear Infections In Your Child is structured to build the reader's knowledge about ear infections. Scattered throughout the text are parents' comments and stories that have been gathered throughout two years of researching and writing. The parents' participation was instrumental in preparing the book: they told us what they wanted to know about otitis media and suggested ways of presenting the information.

Summaries and charts throughout the book are boxed and set off from the text to restate and draw attention to important guidelines and concepts. At the end of each chapter, a question-and-answer format is used to introduce more information about topics covered in that particular chapter. Footnotes are also included at the end of each chapter. Finally, a glossary and index are located at the back of the book.

OTITIS MEDIA IN OUR SOCIETY TODAY ▆▆▆

A Short Look at Otitis Media in History

"To amende deafness, ye shall make an ointment of an hares galle, and the greese or droppings of an ele, which is souerain thyng to recouever hearing."

Remedy for children's earache
in the first English book of
Pediatrics, 1545 by Phaire[1]

Since the age of Hippocrates (460–375 B.C.), and no doubt even earlier, the ear infection has eluded physicians' best efforts to find a cure. Hippocrates, whose writing dominated the medical world for many centuries, apparently was the first to mention the eardrum and describe acute otitis media. But hundreds of years passed before many misconceptions about the anatomy and function of the ear and the eustachian tube were corrected. That lack of knowledge and understanding of the ear led to such bizarre and ineffective treatments as leeches, purgatives, primitive suction of the eustachian tube and removal of the eardrum.

Even as early as 30 B.C., doctors recognized that children had many more ear infections than adults. Celsus (50 B.C.– 10 A.D.) was the first to state that children should be treated differently from adults.

However, it was not until the early 1800s that physicians regularly started treating the ear infection as an open sore by lancing the eardrum with a sharp knife (a procedure now called myringotomy). This was the first major medical breakthrough in relieving the pressure and pain caused by an ear infection. A century later, Adam Politzer introduced the first ventilation tube, although the device wasn't used regularly until 1954.[1]

Though it relieved pain and pressure, myringotomy often did not clear the infection, meaning bacteria could spread from the middle ear and attack the bony structures around the ear and brain. In 1932, otitis media and related serious complications accounted for 27 percent of pediatric admissions to Bellevue Hospital in New York City.[2] More than 4,000 children in the United States died from mastoiditis in 1936 and many others suffered loss of hearing and facial paralysis.[3]

In the early 1940s, the widespread use of antibiotics revolutionized the treatment of ear infection and greatly diminished life-threatening complications. Since then, further strides have been made against this disease: antibiotics are used to curb and control infection; tympanostomy tubes are used to help ventilate the middle ear; and refined instruments for ear examinations and detection of middle ear fluid have resulted in more accurate and more frequent diagnoses of otitis media. Additionally, pediatricians today are better trained in detecting otitis media and they routinely examine children's ears even during well-baby visits.

Otitis Media: A Modern Public Health Problem

Despite these sophisticated methods to diagnose, treat and prevent ear infections, otitis media remains a major public health problem in the United States, with costs for treatment estimated at more than $2 billion annually.[4] It is the most common medical problem for children, and is second only to well-baby visits as the reason for office visits to a pediatrician.[4] One study estimated that one of three children who visit a pediatrician is diagnosed as having an ear infection, and three fourths of follow-up visits were for middle ear disease.[5]

Since the advent of antibiotics, experts have noted that, although life-threatening illness has decreased, the number of children suffering chronic middle ear conditions has increased.[6,7,8] One of the foremost experts in the study of otitis media in the United States is Jack L. Paradise, M.D., Professor of Pediatrics and Community Medicine, University of Pittsburgh School of Medicine, and Medical Director of the Ambulatory Care Center, Children's Hospital of Pittsburgh. Paradise says: "Perhaps we have reduced the number of serious ill-nesses that come from otitis media, but only at the price of increasing the number of patients with chronic disease, which has in turn led to an ever increasing number of surgical pro-cedures to treat and prevent otitis media."[9]

What does this mean in terms of numbers?

- Thirty million visits per year to physicians are estimated to take place for the diagnosis and treatment of otitis media. This includes emergency visits, follow-up visits, consul-tations with ENT specialists, hearing tests and evaluation of speech and language.[4]

- The number of visits for acute care of otitis media is esti-mated to have risen by roughly 58 percent between 1981 and 1987.[10] (See Chart 1.)

- One study estimated that on any one day in the United States, up to 30 percent of children are suffering an ear infection or have an abnormal middle ear condition.[11] That means that up to 900,000 children a day are suffering an ear-related condition in the United States.

- Another survey indicated that, by age one, one-half of the children studied had at least one ear infection; by age three, one-third of the same children had had three or more ear infections.[12]

- Before age six, 90 percent of children in the U.S. will have had at least one ear infection. Half of the children who have one ear infection before the age of one will have six or more episodes in the next two years. Nearly 20 percent of children who suffer ear infections will require, at some time, surgery to correct the problem.[13]

Consequently, researchers are taking a long, hard look at otitis media. They are asking: Are children being overmedi-cated? Are too many children receiving operations too often for treatment of ear infections? What causes chronic otitis media? What children are most at risk? How can otitis media be prevented?

Chart 1

Number of visits to treat acute otitis media
for children under age 9

1981 14,277,000

1987 22,595,000

National Disease and Therapeutic Index (NDTI) Diagnosis Jan.–Dec.
1981 and Jan. 1987–December 1987.

Chart 2

Rate of decrease in number of tonsillectomies
with adenoidectomies in children under age 15

1965 981,000

1975 471,000

1986 144,000

National Hospital Discharge Survey, the National Center for Health
Statistics.

Otitis Media Research

In spite of the prevalence of otitis media among children in
the U.S., researchers admit wide gaps of knowledge exist in
areas as basic as anatomy and physiology of the middle ear
system and eustachian tube. Researchers are studying the
effectiveness of antibiotics and vaccines, the causes of ear
infections, how the immune system plays a role in preventing

otitis media and the most effective methods to manage chronic conditions.

At least three major hospital centers in the United States are conducting extensive research into the causes, management and treatment of otitis media. The National Institutes of Health has funded three otitis media research centers: at the University of Minnesota in 1978; at the Children's Hospital of Pittsburgh in 1980; and at the Children's Hospital in Boston in 1986.

These centers draw upon the expertise of scientists, practitioners and educators from many fields and encourage work between the practicing physician and the scientist. For instance, microbiologists, anatomists, biophysicians, biostatiticians and experts in public health and infectious disease all work together on research projects. The Otitis Media Research Center in Boston involves experts from Boston City Hospital, Harvard University, Boston University School of Education and pediatric clinics and private practices. This collaboration symbolizes the diverse impact that otitis media has on many areas of health.

Research in otitis media is also being conducted at other universities in the United States. This research is not only being funded through the federal government, at an estimated cost of nearly $6 million in 1988,[14] but through public corporations and private companies such as equipment manufacturers and pharmaceutical companies.

The Economics of Otitis Media

The relationship between patient and physician is changing as dramatically as the society in which we live. The general practitioner was once a trusted friend who may have treated several generations of one family. A visit with a doctor, who often made house calls, was often as much a social interaction as a means for providing medical care. Today, each family member may have his or her own physician, depending on age and need, and may consult two or three physicians for a serious illness. Or, the family may belong to a group health plan in which family members see a different doctor every time they attend a clinic.

The treatment of your child is no doubt affected by the increasing economic pressures felt by your physician. In 1986, there were 216 physicians for every 100,000 Americans;[15] by 2000, that number is expected to reach 249.[15] This growing surplus of physicians and the spiraling cost of malpractice insurance have forced the medical profession to confront the same economic realities faced by any business: The physician in private practice today must contend with increased overhead expenses and must compete with group health plans, plans that provide for reduced fees for patients, and colleagues developing innovative ways to "keep" their patients.

A doctor's diagnoses and referrals also may be directly influenced by incentives given by hospitals and medical insurance policies. Hospitals are beginning to evaluate physicians' surgery practices and fee schedules and penalize doctors whom they believe perform unnecessary surgery or charge excessive fees.

Physicians are loathe to admit that financial pressures influence their decision-making; nonetheless, these financial pressures must have *some* impact upon the way treatment is chosen. In treatment of otitis media, millions of dollars are at stake: drug companies send free samples to physicians to encourage use of their antibiotics; experts receive grant money from manufacturers to test medications; pediatricians may hesitate to make referrals to otolaryngologists for fear of losing patients; otolaryngologists may be inclined to recommend surgical procedures, the costs of which are fully covered by insurance policies.

The complex interplay among these economic and social forces is no simple matter to interpret; but parents should be aware of the many social and economic factors that can affect the treatment of the decision-making process that takes place when children are being treated for otitis media. These forces often contribute to a course of treatment that is so rigid or routine that a physician never deviates from one patient to the next. For instance, a physician may automatically prescribe antibiotics without a thorough ear examination. Or he may state unequivocably that tubes are wrong for all children. Or the specialist may declare immediately that your child "must have tubes." These inflexible and unyielding attitudes may indicate that the physician is not evaluating your child as an individual.

Costs of Otitis Media

The total yearly costs related to management of otitis media in the United States have been estimated to be as high as $2 billion,[4] which include costs for doctors' visits, surgery, medications and referrals and tests by audiologists and speech-language pathologists.

What does this mean for the individual family? One survey estimated that, in 1985, a family spent $90 on medical costs for each episode of otitis media.[16] Charts 3, 4, and 5 give examples of specific costs, though the hidden costs of transportation and time lost from work are impossible to determine. A family that is covered by health insurance will probably continue to seek the best care for its children, at whatever cost. But what about the family whose health care is not reimbursed by an insurance plan? Many of these families probably would have to restrict their children's medical care because of financial considerations.

Charts 6, 7, and 8 are based on results from the National Medical Expenditure Survey conducted in 1977 and show how costs associated with otitis media have risen in the past eight years. It is expected that, when the newest survey results are available in 1989, the increase in costs will be much more dramatic than shown in the charts because the 1985 figures have been adjusted for inflation and do not reflect the increase in the number of children being treated for otitis media.

Chart 3

Average costs of medication used to treat otitis media

Nonprescription

Tylenol®
Sudafed® $4 for
Dimetapp®   4 fluid oz.
Actifed®

Prescription

Amoxicillin—$8.80
Septra®—$9.95
Bactrim®—$9.75
Ceclor®—$46   10-day
Gantrisin®—$9.75   supply
Augmentin®—$41
Pediazole®—$32

Tylenol® with codeine—$12.75 for 4 oz.
Cortisporin Otic® (eardrops)—$21 for 5-day supply
Auralgan® (eardrops)—$10 for 5-day supply

Chart 4

Average costs of doctor's visits, consultations, tests

Pediatrician: acute office visit = $25
Pediatrician: follow-up visit = $21
ENT specialist: consultation = $35–$50
ENT specialist: myringotomy = $100
Audiologist: hearing test = $60–$90
Speech-language pathologist: evaluation = $120

Chart 5

Costs for Insertion of Ear Tubes
In Doctor's Office:*
  Surgeon's fees—one ear = $200
         Two ears = $250

In Operating Room:*
  Surgeon's fees for one ear = $280
        two ears = $490
  Anesthesiologist's fees—$400
  Medical and surgical supplies ⎫
  Laboratory tests   ⎬ $600
  Anesthesiologist materials ⎭
  Drugs from pharmacy
  Operating room and recovery room = $350

*Costs are averages of 3 major children's hospitals in United States.

Social Forces Affecting Otitis Media

Part of the apparent rise in ear infections among our children may be attributed to fundamental changes in our society. The increasing number of families with two working parents has led to more and younger infants in day care centers. These children, who easily spread disease among themselves, are at risk of developing an ear infection with every exposure to colds or respiratory infection.[17,18]

In addition, many working parents don't have the time to stay home and take care of their children—they seek a "quick fix" for their child so they can get back to work. This is not only the fault of the parent, but also the fault of a society in which employers can be insensitive to the needs of working parents and the stress that a child's illness places on a family.

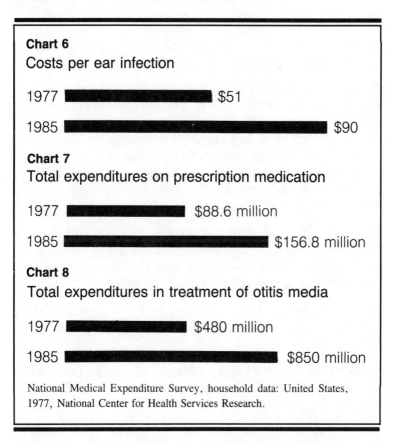

Chart 6
Costs per ear infection

1977 $51

1985 $90

Chart 7
Total expenditures on prescription medication

1977 $88.6 million

1985 $156.8 million

Chart 8
Total expenditures in treatment of otitis media

1977 $480 million

1985 $850 million

National Medical Expenditure Survey, household data: United States, 1977, National Center for Health Services Research.

This "quick fix" often takes the form of antibiotic treatment. Most parents believe that antibiotics are a quick "cure" for infection—and any parent, working or not, wants their child to be given the best treatment available—the one that is going to relieve pain in the least amount of time. But for the child with chronic ear problems, there is no magical cure. Often, a reasonable remedy for a child is to stay home and rest for a couple of days when a cold or earache develops. This demands time and patience on the part of today's busy parents.

The Impact of Ear Infections on Families

A family with a child who has recurrent ear problems often has its routine disrupted. For example:

Medication. The sick child has to be given antibiotics three or four times a day for 10 days. Does the parent remember to faithfully administer the right dosage at the right times every day? Some children spit out the medicine or struggle when the medicine is given to them. Can the parent be sure that the child received the right amount? If the child is in day care, can the parent be sure that the caretakers remember to administer the correct dosage?

Travel plans. Making travel plans can be difficult because the child can be well one day and sick the next or may not be able to fly at the appointed time. And there's always the possibility the child will fall ill away from home.

Sleepless nights. Many nights of broken sleep cause short tempers and further susceptibility to illness for family members.

Trips to the doctor's office. Children who suffer many bouts of otitis media spend much time in doctor's offices for initial treatment of the infection and for follow-up visits. This means that a parent must devote an inordinate amount of time making appointments, driving back and forth to the physician's office, juggling schedules of other family members, and perhaps taking time off from work. This time in the doctor's office also disrupts a child's normal schedule that is better spent socializing with peers or spending a normal day with the primary caretaker.

The guilty and anxious parent. Many parents worry about the cause of the chronic ear infection; and this worrying often turns into frustration or bewilderment as the parent talks with other parents whose doctors often have recommended a completely different course of treatment.

Ultimately, many parents blame themselves for the chronic illnesses because there seems to be no other place to lay the blame. A sense of helplessness can overcome a parent who watches her child suffer pain again and again, and whose own stamina is worn down by lack of sleep and anxiety. Additionally, for the parent of an infant or toddler, the stress is heightened by the child's inability to verbalize his or her pain. The parent is continually guessing as to whether a bit of fussiness or a pulling at an ear means the child is suffering ear pain or is just having a bad day.

The Emotional Health of Your Child

Some of the above problems may affect your family throughout the time your child is suffering chronic ear problems. How will your family and your child react to these different stresses?

Many parents allow their child's illness to dominate their family's lives. They fear they are spoiling their child when he is healthy (to compensate for the times he is sick); they fear the child demands and becomes accustomed to the special treatment he receives when ill. Certainly, this can lead to resentment and anger toward a child—feelings that most children will notice.

Other parents begin to read signs of illness into every facet of the child's behavior or health. For instance, a common frustration for parents of children under age 2 is that they can't tell if cranky and fussy symptoms mean the child has an ear infection, if he's hungry or sleepy, if he's cutting teeth, or if he's just in a grumpy mood. Obviously, it's easy to assign the blame to an ear infection and rush him to the doctor for another prescription of antibiotics. As the child gets older, the ear infection can still be used as an excuse for hyperactivity, inattentiveness, emotional immaturity or poor school performance. Certainly, recurrent ear infections can affect a child's behavior. But parents must realize their children go through emotional highs and lows throughout their development that result in good days and bad days (or good weeks and bad weeks). Parents should try to keep the impact of ear infections in perspective—it is only one of the multiple and complex forces that shape a child's behavior and personality.

Any of these concerns could be a legitimate cause for further discussion between parents or between parents and physician. Often, a physician, or a more experienced parent or grandparent can put into better perspective a problem that isn't as overwhelming as it seems to young and anxious parents. In fact, many times the parents are more upset about a child's recurrent illnesses than the child is. Most children are extremely adaptable to their lifestyle: they'll take up where they left off before they were sick and jump into the thick of life with little recall that they just spent three days in bed, or just underwent minor surgery to have tubes put in their ears.

Events surrounding an illness should never be ignored, but certainly those events shouldn't be made the focus of a child's life. When healthy, the child should be given every opportunity to enjoy his days as every other child would: spending time with his parents and siblings, exploring his environment, playing with other children, eating dinner with the family. These are the simple, routine, everyday activities that give a child emotional happiness and health.

NOTES ━━━━━━━━━━━━━━━━━━━━━━━━━━━━━━━━

1.   Pahor AL. An Early History of Secretory Otitis Media. The Journal of Laryngology and Otology. 1978 July: 543–560.

2.   Klein JO. "Antimicrobial Management and Prevention of Otitis Media with Effusion" in Recent Advances in Otitis Media with Effusion (DJ Lim, Editor in Chief). B.C. Decker Inc., 1984:276–277.

3.   Wright PF. Indication and Duration of Antimicrobial Agents for Acute Otitis Media. Pediatric Annals. 1984 May: 13 (5): 377–379.

4.   Bluestone CD. Otitis Media: Update 1984. Infectious Diseases. 1984 April: 14(4): 4.

5.   Teele DW, Klein JO, Rosner B, et al. Middle Ear Disease and the Practice of Pediatrics: Burden During the First Five Years of Life. JAMA. 1983: 249:1026.

6.   Paparella MM, Schachern PA. "Complications and Sequelae

of Otitis Media: State of the Art" in Recent Advances in Otitis Media with Effusion (DJ Lim, Editor in Chief). B.C. Decker Inc., 1984: 316–319.

7. Gates GA. "Management" in Recent Advances in Otitis Media With Effusion (Lim DJ, editor). Annals of Otology, Rhinol and Laryngol. 1985 Jan–Feb: Suppl 116, 94 (1;3) 27–30.

8. Shambaugh GE. "Complications of Otitis Media" in Otitis Media: Publication of the Second National Conference on Otitis Media (RJ Wiet and SW Coulthard, coeditors). 1979, Ross Laboratories: 48–50.

9. Bluestone CD (moderator). "Panel Discussion: Controversies in Antimicrobial Therapy for Otitis Media" in Recent Advances in Otitis Media with Effusion (DJ Lim, Editor in Chief). B.C. Decker Inc., 1984: 290–292.

10. National Disease and Therapeutic Index (NDTI), Diagnosis, Jan–Dec. 1984 and Jan–Dec 1987.

11. Jerger, JF. "Dissenting Report: Mass Impedance Screening" in Recent Advances in Otitis Media With Effusion (Lim DJ, editor). Ann Otol Rhinol Laryngol. 1980 May–June; 89 (Suppl 69) (3)(3): 21–22.

12. Teele DW, Klein JO, Rosner B. Epidemiology of Otitis Media in Children. Ann Otol Rhinol Laryngol May–June 1980; 89 (Suppl 68): 5–6.

13. Paparella MM, Juhn SK. "Otitis Media: Definitions and Terminology" in Otitis Media: Proceedings of the Second National Conference on Otitis Media (co-editors RJ Wiet and SW Coulthard). 1979 January; Ross Laboratories, Columbus Ohio; 2–8.

14. Information based on list of CRISP records of currently active USPHS grants and contracts and NIH intramural projects active in 1988 from the Division of Research Grants, Department of Health and Human Services, Public Health Service.

15. Sixth report to the President and Congress on the Status of Health Personnel in the U.S. DHHS. Public Health Service.

16. National Medical Expenditure Survey, household data: United States, 1977. National Center for Health Services Research.

17. B Vinther, Pedersen B, Elbrond O. "Otitis Media in Childhood. Sociomedical Aspects with Special Reference to Day-Care Situations." Clin Otolaryngol. 1984 Feb: 9 (1): 3–8.

18. B Vinther, Elbrond O. "A Population Study of Otitis Media in Childhood." Acto Otolaryngol (Stockh) Suppl 360:135, 1979.

PART ONE

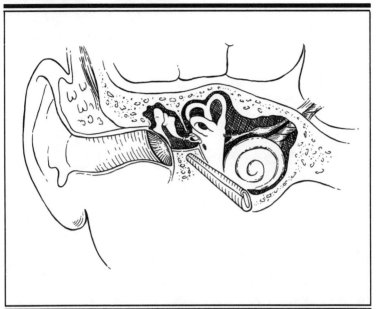

Medical Facts About Ear Infections

CHAPTER ONE

Mechanics of the Ear

A parent has rushed her feverish and lethargic six-month-old daughter to the doctor's office for an ear examination. The ill child cries at the sight of a stranger and screams at the touch of the ear-examining instrument. As the sobbing child clings to her mother, the doctor puts down his instrument, looks at the parent very seriously, and says, "Yes, it definitely looks like acute otitis media. Her tympanic membrane is bulging with what appears to be purulent effusion, and that is probably what has caused the otalgia. Let's try a myringotomy for now, and I'll prescribe either amoxicillin or Bactrim®."

After straining to listen to this explanation over the cries of a child, some parents would be so bewildered and exasperated that they wouldn't bother to ask questions; others would lose their tempers and demand an explanation in lay terms. The doctor could avoid these reactions by stating instead: "Yes, it looks like your child has a severe ear infection. There is thick fluid in the middle ear that is bulging against the eardrum and causing ear pain. Let's lance the eardrum for now and I'll prescribe antibiotics that will help the infection clear up."

Even doctors who are very good at explaining medical conditions to patients will use terms that sound like Greek or Latin—which is understandable, since those are the languages

23

from which most medical language is derived. Parents who admit they don't understand the physician's language or terminology are in a good position to discuss their child's problems with a physician. Politely interrupt your physician if you don't understand him. Most physicians take this as a cue to simplify their explanations. If you're still confused, ask the doctor to explain the situation in lay terms.

Parents equipped with background about medical terminology are less confused and intimidated by the words the doctor uses. Many medical terms can be more easily remembered, understood and pronounced when parents understand they are built of parts that, when put together, add up to mean the whole. For instance, otitis media can be broken into three Greek root words: ot–ear; itis–inflammation; media–middle. Otitis media means inflammation of the middle ear. Otalgia, or earache, can be broken into two Greek root words: ot–ear; algia–pain. The glossary at the end of the book includes root words to help readers better understand the meaning of medical terms.

INSIDE THE EAR ═══════════════════════════

The ear is divided into three parts—called the outer, middle and inner ear—and is capable of receiving, amplifying and transmitting hundreds of thousands of tones rapidly and efficiently to the brain, which interprets sound.

The only part of this organ visible is what we commonly call the "ear," but what is described in anatomical terms as the auricle or pinna. Directly inside the auricle is the ear canal, known as the external auditory canal. This canal is sealed at its inner end by the eardrum, or tympanic membrane, which is a broad, flat, cone-shaped membrane about one half-inch in diameter and less than 1/50th of an inch thick. The eardrum is similar to wax paper: it is very delicate and sensitive, and appears brilliantly translucent under the light of a physician's examining instrument. *By observing changes in the eardrum*

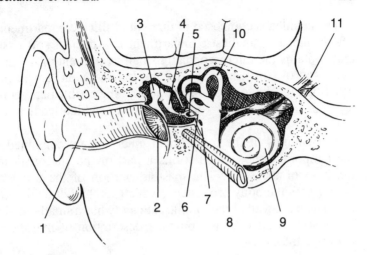

Anatomy of the ear:

1) External canal
2) Eardrum
   (tympanic membrane)
3) Malleus
4) Incus
5) Stapes

6) Oval window
7) Round window
8) Eustachian tube
9) Cochlea
10) Semicircular canal
11) Auditory nerve

such as appearance, color, position and mobility, the physician determines if there is fluid in the middle ear.

The three tiniest bones in the body, collectively called the ossicles, are the malleus, incus and stapes (or the hammer, anvil and stirrup). They form a bridge that connects the eardrum with the oval window, an opening in the wall of the middle ear that leads to the inner ear. The foot of the stapes rests on the oval window. Beyond the oval window lies the inner ear, a snail-shaped chamber filled with fluid. The lower part of the inner ear is the spiral-shaped cochlea. It is about the size of a fingertip. The central and upper sections of the chamber contain the body's balance mechanism and do not contribute to the hearing mechanism.

The cochlea is composed of three fluid-filled compartments. The center and smallest compartment is a duct of soft tissue that contains the microscopically small instrument of hearing, the organ of Corti, named after the Italian scientist who first described it. Nerve fibers spiral around the cochlea and come together in the auditory (or eighth) nerve, which leads to the brain.

The cavities of the middle and inner ear are contained in the temporal bone, which forms a part of the side wall and the base of the skull. The mastoid portion of the temporal bone forms the bony prominence which can be felt behind the ear. The back wall of the middle ear cavity has a small opening onto mastoid air cells (a complete description of mastoiditis is on Page 92).

Membranes in the Middle Ear

The lining inside the nose, nasopharynx, eustachian tube and middle air space is composed of many different kinds of cells that perform varying functions. Two types of cells that play an important role in middle ear function are mucus-producing cells called goblet cells, and the cells that move mucus, cilliated cells. Cilia are short, hairlike outgrowths of certain cells that move substances with a rhythmic, beating action. In the middle ear, the cilia moves mucus or fluid into the eustachian tube and in the eustachian tube and nose, cilia moves mucus or fluid into the nasopharynx.

In order for the cells in the middle ear to thrive, they must be "fed" the oxygen supplied when the eustachian tube opens. If the eustachian tube is blocked or not opening and closing properly, the cells absorb the remaining oxygen and a vacuum can be created.

When Sound Enters the Ear Canal

The outer ear collects and intercepts sound and channels it into the ear canal. The sound energy is amplified by the ear canal, which doubles the pressure of certain sounds in the range humans hear best.

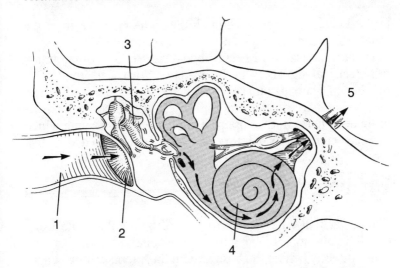

When sound enters the ear canal, (1) it strikes and causes the eardrum to vibrate (2). The vibrations are sent through the ossicles (3) and into the cochlea (4), which transmits a signal to the brain via the auditory nerve (5).

As the sound waves strike the eardrum, vibrations are transmitted to the ossicles, which in turn vibrate the inner ear fluid. In order for these vibrations to occur, the ossicular chain must be surrounded by air; *if fluid fills the middle ear space, the effectiveness of the mechanical action of the chain of bones can be greatly reduced because sound energy is not well transformed into mechanical energy.*

The tiny ossicles, tripling the incoming sound pressure, converts airborne sound energy from the outer ear to mechanical energy in the middle ear. Sound pressure is then amplified 30 times as it becomes concentrated on the oval window (which is 1/30th the surface area of the eardrum).

As the stapes vibrates in the oval window, its footplate bulges against the inner ear and sends sound waves swelling through the cochlear fluid. This is where the organ of Corti plays its part. Inside this microscopically small organ are about 24,000 specialized touch cells, known as "hair" cells, which "feel" movements of the fluid and stimulate the nerve fibers to send electrical signals through the auditory nerve from the inner ear to the hearing center in the brain.

It takes thousands of nerve fibers—about 25,000—to transmit electrical signals from the organ of Corti. The greater the number of fibers a sound activates, the louder the sound. The nerve signals reach the brain as an electrical code which the brain deciphers. But the brain can only decipher a sound which has been stored in its memory. An adult's brain can distinguish almost 400,000 different sounds.

THE EUSTACHIAN TUBE

The eustachian tube is a narrow canal with collapsible walls that links the middle ear with the nasopharynx, which is the space directly behind the nose. About the thickness of a pencil, the eustachian tube opens hundreds of times a day, usually with every third swallow and with every yawn. When the tube opens, air enters the canal and travels to the middle ear.

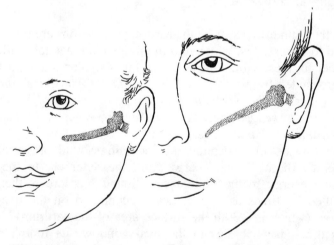

With growth, the eustachian tube becomes more vertical and its cartilage becomes stiffer. A child's eustachian tube is less able than an adult's to drain fluid efficiently and close and open efficiently.

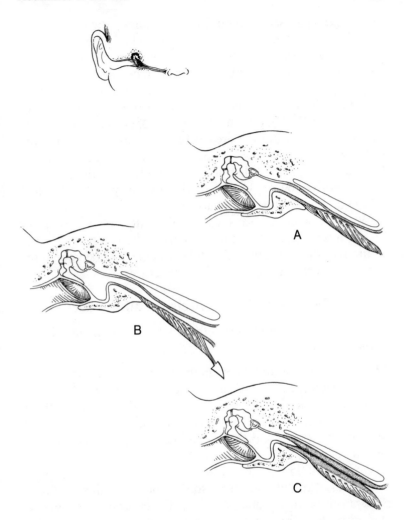

The eustachian tube (top) is a passageway for air to the middle ear and a drainage path for fluid from the middle ear to the throat. In "A", the eustachian tube is closed in its resting state. In "B", the eustachian tube opens as the person swallows. The arrow shows the muscle contracting to pull open the tube. In "C", the eustachian tube is not able to open because the inside lining of the tube is swollen.

A child's eustachian tube differs in shape, angle and structure from an adult's. A child's eustachian tube is shorter, wider, more horizontal and more compliant or "floppy." This "immaturity" of the eustachian tube can be one of the reasons why children have more frequent ear infections than adults. The eustachian tube may contribute to otitis media in three ways: (1) the "floppy" tube remains open and allows substances to pass from the area behind the nose (nasopharynx) to the middle ear (this is called a "patent" eustachian tube); (2) the tube becomes obstructed or swollen; (3) the tube is at such a horizontal angle that fluid does not pass easily from the middle ear to the nasopharynx.

When your doctor says your child will probably outgrow his ear infections when he reaches age 4, he is referring partly to the fact that the eustachian tube's angle will become more vertical and its cartilage will become stiffer.

How the Eustachian Tube Protects the Middle Ear

The eustachian tube performs three vital functions in relation to the middle ear:

1) The eustachian tube's opening and closing mechanism allows the middle ear to "breathe." Scientists call this the "ventilation" function of the eustachian tube. When the eustachian tube is swollen shut or is blocked, the cells within the middle ear absorb oxygen and the middle ear space can become an airless vacuum.

This ventilation function also helps to equalize air pressure in the closed middle ear space so that the same air pressure is present on the inside and outside of the eardrum. This equalization protects your middle ear from harmful pressure differences that can occur in a fast-rising elevator, for example, or on takeoff and landing in an airplane. That's why chewing gum or swallowing relieves the stuffiness in your ear during airplane travel—swallowing opens the eustachian tube and allows middle ear pressure to equalize with atmospheric pressure.

2) The eustachian tube is like a drainage tube for the middle ear; if fluid starts to build up within the middle ear, the eustachian tube provides a pathway for clearance of fluid from the middle ear to the throat (nasopharynx).

3) The eustachian tube protects the middle ear from substances, such as bacteria, viruses or particles, blown into the nasopharynx when a child blows his nose, sniffs, sneezes or coughs.

The Eustachian Tube

Function

1) Ventilates middle ear
2) Allows fluid to drain into throat
3) Protects middle ear from substances blown through throat

Malfunction

1) "Floppy" tube does not close properly
2) Tube becomes obstructed or swollen
3) Tube's angle doesn't allow fluid to drain

OTHER STRUCTURES THAT CAN AFFECT MIDDLE EAR FUNCTION

Adenoids and Tonsils: Adenoids are growths of lymphoid tissue in the upper part of the throat, behind the nose. The tonsils are a pair of oval masses of lymphoid tissue, one on each side of the throat at the back of the mouth. The tonsils and adenoids, especially in childhood, can become infected and swollen. Researchers have speculated that the infected tissue can play a role in childhood ear infections in two ways: the bacteria or

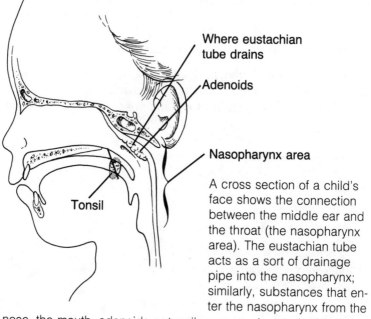

Where eustachian tube drains

Adenoids

Nasopharynx area

Tonsil

A cross section of a child's face shows the connection between the middle ear and the throat (the nasopharynx area). The eustachian tube acts as a sort of drainage pipe into the nasopharynx; similarly, substances that enter the nasopharynx from the nose, the mouth, adenoids or tonsils can crawl up or be blown into the eustachian tube and enter the middle ear.

virus can spread from the infected tissue to the middle ear via the eustachian tube; or the adenoids can swell up and block the eustachian tube. (See discussion of adenoidectomy on page 125.)

Palate: The eustachian tube always remains closed until opened by the pull of muscles attached to the roof of the mouth, called the palate. During swallowing and yawning, the muscles from the palate to the eustachian tube contract and the tube opens. Any defect of the soft or hard palate, such as a cleft palate, can prevent the eustachian tube from opening and closing efficiently. (See discussion of cleft palate on pages 45–46.)

INFECTION: INVASION AND DEFENSE ━━━

What Is Infection?

Our bodies are inhabited by millions of small organisms, called microorganisms or microbes, that cannot be seen without the aid of magnification. Microbes are found on our skin, in our noses, in our intestines, in our food. Normally, these microorganisms live in harmony with our bodies.

Disease and infection occur when microorganisms (called pathogens) move into a part of the body where they are not normally situated; when they invade body tissues that are normally germ-free; or when they produce poisonous substances that damage the surrounding microbes or body tissues.

Two types of microorganisms that can cause middle ear infection are known as bacteria and viruses. Pathogens that can cause respiratory disease are often passed directly by infected individuals through sneezing, coughing or touching, or even on drinking glasses or eating utensils. Once the pathogens enter the respiratory tract, they feed and multiply on nutrients supplied by body fluids and thrive in the warm temperature of the body.

Once the respiratory tract is invaded by bacteria or virus, its mucous membranes and other cells react by swelling and creating extra mucus to fight the invasion. *Many children commonly suffer an ear infection after the symptoms of a cold start to subside because bacteria invade the nose during or after the viral infection and the bacteria "crawl up" through the eustachian tube into the middle ear.*

Once the bacteria enter the middle ear, the lining of the middle ear secretes extra mucus to fight the invasion. If the eustachian tube is not obstructed, this accumulated fluid may drain through the tube and the infection may clear up without any signs of ear pain. But if the eustachian tube is obstructed, or is not opening and closing properly, then infected fluid can accumulate and bulge against, or even rupture, the eardrum.

How the Body Fights Infection

After invasion of bacteria or virus, the body mounts a defense, called the immune response, that can contribute both to recovery from the illness and to protection against reinfection.

Once the dangerous microbe gets beyond the body's first line of defense (the skin and mucous membrane), the cellular system of the body comes to the rescue. In short, blood flow to the infected area is increased and special blood cells are sent to the area. These special cells can surround and ingest the bacteria, virus or other foreign material. The last line of defense of the body is the creation of antibodies to fight the disease. This type of immunity occurs either naturally (such as when a child gets the chicken pox and can never get it again), or when a serum is injected into the blood (such as a diphtheria-pertussis-whooping cough (DPT) vaccination).

Scientists have found that a local immune system in the middle ear produces specific antibodies to bacteria that cause ear infection.[1] If these antibodies are present during an infection, they can help clear the middle ear of fluid and restore it to a normal state. However, the creation of these antibodies does not necessarily prevent a recurrent infection, but may help reduce the duration of the middle ear fluid.

Although much is known about the fundamental processes of natural immunity, very little is understood. Sometimes our immune system can prevent an invasion of a dangerous microorganism, sometimes it is helpless to fight the pathogen. Factors such as nutrition, illness, physical stress and heredity affect the workings of the immune system. (For more discussion of the immune system, see page 48.)

Many parents whose children are healthy and robust are distraught by the recurrence of ear infections, despite their attempts to guard their children from fatigue and poor diet. The study of immunology in the role of ear infections is a new area of investigation. Perhaps in the coming years, when scientists focus on the middle ear's system of fighting infection, more answers will be found to help parents prevent their children from suffering ear infections.

QUESTIONS AND ANSWERS ━━━━━━

Q: Can an ear infection spread from one ear to the other?

A: Not really. The nose and nasopharynx may harbor bacteria and viruses that can cause ear infections. Sometimes bacteria from the nasopharynx will reach one ear before the other ear is affected. However, there is no scientific evidence to support the notion that infection can spread from one ear to another. One ear can be more susceptible if the eustachian tube on that side does not function as well as the eustachian tube on the other side.

Q: If my child has an infection in both ears, could different bacteria be causing the problem?

A: Yes. However, there is no way to tell exactly which bacteria are causing the infection without removing fluid from each ear and culturing the fluid.

NOTE ━━━━━━

1. Bluestone CD, Klein JO. "Otitis Media with Effusion, Atelectasis and Eustachian Tube Dysfunction" in Pediatric Otolaryngology Volume 1 (edited by CD Bluestone and SE Stool). 1983 WB Saunders Co.: 410.

CHAPTER TWO

Defining Otitis Media

E ffective communication depends on a common understanding of the meaning of words. Does "otitis media" mean the same to you as it does to your doctor, or your spouse, or another parent? You may define it as ear infection; but if you ask three different people to define ear infection, you will get three different answers.

"Otitis media" and "ear infection" are words that convey different meanings and are associated with a myriad of emotions and mysteries. For many parents, the words "otitis media" evoke feelings of anxiety because an ear infection is a disease in a tiny and hidden part of the body that causes severe pain and dramatic symptoms in young, vulnerable children. Others are frightened by a disease they believe can lead to a life threatening illness or to deafness.

The problem of defining otitis media is a concern even among physicians who gather regularly to report on the most recent research and advances concerning ear infections. Because so many researchers around the world are studying various aspects of otitis media, an international panel of experts has developed standard definitions of otitis media. Knowing that their definitions may not always be followed, the experts urged researchers to define the disease they are studying or describing.[1]

Another group of researchers queried seven leading otolaryngologists in the country and asked them questions including: what constitutes an episode of otitis media and what is its duration? Because of the diverse and sometimes conflicting replies, the researchers stated: ''There seems to be no scientific data or guidelines for defining an episode of otitis media . . . we conclude that it would be a valuable contribution of some group to propose a definition of otitis media.''[2]

This attempt at standardization may be useful to researchers and experts, but physicians must use these terms on a daily basis with parents who may already have fearful associations and incorrect meanings attached to the term ''otitis media.'' Parents derive these meanings from child-care books, from friends and relatives, and even from physicians.

The Importance of Understanding What Otitis Media Means

Why is it so important for a parent to know what a doctor means when he says a child has ''otitis media''? First and foremost, the diagnosis of otitis media determines the treatment. Ask your doctor what he means when he says ''otitis media.'' Does he mean infected fluid is bulging against the eardrum and causing pain? Does he mean he sees fluid bubbles but doesn't detect any inflammation? The first condition most probably warrants medication and possibly lancing of the eardrum; the second condition can probably be left untreated.

Second, the doctor's meaning of ''otitis media'' may create an emotional response within the parent. Does this mean my child is seriously ill? If so, the parent's anxiety and concern may be perceived by the child, possibly making the child feel worse. Conversely, a parent and child will be much more at ease with the condition if the doctor says it's a very natural and normal childhood occurrence that will resolve quickly and with no ill effects.

One mother of an eight-month-old child, who was referred to an ENT specialist by a pediatrician, was very anxious about her child's ear problems. She told the specialist that the child had been on antibiotics for many months because of "an ear infection that would not go away." When the specialist asked her what the child's symptoms had been for the past two months, the mother replied that the child had seemed fine most of the time. However, she said that every time she took the baby in for a follow-up examination, the pediatrician told her the "ear infection" had not gone away. Upon examination, the specialist determined that the child had some fluid in the ear and explained the difference between an acute ear infection and persistent middle ear fluid. The mother told the specialist that she had been very upset about the child's condition because she thought the child had been sick with an "ear infection" for many months and was uneasy about possible consequences.

Definitions Used in This Book

The terms defined below are used throughout the book, and in many places, the definitions are repeated.

Definitions of Otitis Media

Acute otitis media: Inflammation of eardrum

Middle ear fluid: Noninfected fluid collects in middle ear

Middle ear ventilation disorder: Retracted eardrum

Persistent middle ear fluid: Fluid for 10 weeks or more

Frequently occurring acute otitis media: 4 or more ear infections in 2 consecutive seasons

---

The first three definitions describe conditions that will usually resolve spontaneously or with medical treatment. The last two conditions are often described by physicians as being "chronic." We chose not to use the word "chronic," however, because it incorrectly implies the condition cannot be cured.

Acute otitis media: Rapid and immediate onset of signs and symptoms of infection in the middle ear means infected fluid is pressing against the eardrum and probably causing ear pain. One or more of the following may be present: ear pain, fever, irritability. This condition is sometimes called purulent or suppurative otitis media.

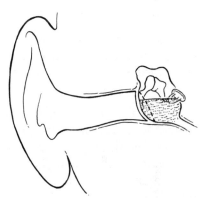

The dotted line shows the normal position of the eardrum. In this depiction of otitis media, the infected fluid is bulging and stretching the eardrum's delicate and tender membrane, resulting in an "earache."

Middle ear fluid: The presence of fluid in the middle ear, usually causing no distress or symptoms, is often called "effusion" by doctors. After the acute symptoms of an ear infection have passed, fluid commonly lingers in the middle ear for many weeks and sometimes months. From 50 to 70 percent of children have middle ear fluid after an acute ear infection;[3,4] a month after an infection, 40 percent still have fluid; two months later, 20 percent have fluid; four months later, five percent have fluid.[3]

Three types of fluid can be present in the ear: serous is a thin, watery fluid; purulent is a yellowish pus-like fluid; mucoid is a thick, viscid, mucuslike fluid.

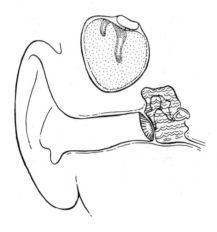

The middle ear cavity is full of fluid that has accumulated after an acute infection. The top drawing shows what the physician would see if he was looking at the eardrum through an otoscope.

Middle ear fluid is described in various ways: some doctors call it otitis media with effusion; others secretory or serous otitis media. Some doctors term any fluid observed in the ear as an "ear infection."

Middle ear ventilation disorder: No fluid and only mild or intermittent discomfort is present in this condition. When severe, the eardrum can be drawn into the middle ear space and cannot move back and forth in response to the physician's examining instrument. When this occurs, a doctor may observe that the eardrum is "retracted" or sucked in. This condition

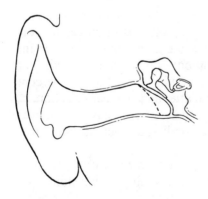

In the retracted state, the eardrum is sucked into the middle ear cavity. Above, the dotted line shows where the eardrum is usually present.

is caused by ''negative pressure'' pulling the eardrum into the middle ear space. This negative pressure is usually present because the middle ear space has developed a vacuum and is not being ventilated properly by the eustachian tube.

Persistent middle ear fluid: The presence of fluid in an ear for more than 10 weeks.

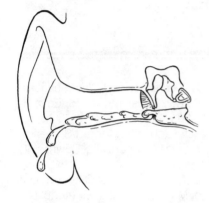

This drawing shows fluid draining from the ear after an eardrum has ruptured.

Frequently occurring acute otitis media: More than three episodes of acute otitis media in each of two consecutive seasons (for instance, four infections in fall, then five infections in winter). Many physicians refer to this condition as chronic otitis media.

Outer Ear Infection

A definition of outer ear infection (otitis externa) is included in this chapter to help parents understand the difference between outer and middle ear conditions and because ''swimmer's ear''—an outer ear infection—is such a common occurrence among children.

Water trapped in the ear canal, especially during hot, humid weather, creates an environment favorable to bacterial or fungal growth that can multiply quickly and irritate the skin of the ear canal. This irritation can lead to painful inflammation of the skin that will itch and may become full of pus.

Over-the-counter ear drops or ear plugs can be used to help lessen the chances of this condition in children who swim often. However, if a child's outer ear becomes infected, he may have to be treated by a physician, who will clean the ear to remove all debris and then instruct the patient to cleanse the ear and apply ear drops daily.

NOTES ═══════════════════════════════════

1.   Bluestone CD. "State of the Art: Definitions and Classifications" in Recent Advances in Otitis Media with Effusion (DJ Lim, Editor in Chief). B.C. Decker Inc., 1984: 1–4.

2.   Personal communication. Bulletin and letter, Project/Screening Children for Communication Disorders. Northern JL, Downs MP, Walker D. 1985 Sept 4.

3.   Teele DW, Klein JO, Rosner B. Epidemiology of Otitis Media in Children. Ann Otol Rhinol Laryngol May–June 1980; 89 (suppl 68): 5–6.

4.   Schwartz RH, Rodriguez WJ, Grundfast KM. Duration of middle ear effusion after acute otitis media. Pediatric Infectious Disease. 1984, Williams and Wilkins Co.: 204–227.

CHAPTER THREE

Causes of Ear Infections

Even the most experienced doctor can have occasional difficulty finding the cause of a child's recurrent ear infections. Of all the parts of the body, a child's middle ear is the most susceptible to infection. Many factors can contribute to a child's recurrent ear infections, and some of those factors may not be easy to pinpoint. Consequently, attempts to answer the question, "Why does my child get so many ear infections?" have consumed countless hours of research by experts studying otitis media.

When discussing with her doctor reasons for her child's third ear infection, one mother said she was insulted because the doctor said, "Some kids are just prone to ear infections. We don't know why."

"I thought he was trying to dodge my question, or that he didn't think I could possibly understand the causes of ear infections," the mother said. Another answer which bristles many parents is: "Children are just sick a lot. It's not uncommon for a child to have a runny nose and several ear infections throughout the winter season."

In fact, it *is* common for most children to suffer three to four ear infections during the winter season, along with seemingly endless runny noses and coughs. The physician who responds with vague answers to your questions about the cause of your child's ear infections may be giving you the most honest answer he can.

If your child is suffering frequently occurring otitis media, however, the doctor should begin the sometimes difficult task of determining the cause. Often, many factors play a role in otitis media—some preventable, others anatomical, and some hereditary. Determining the cause can help the physician find the best treatment for your child.

WHO GETS EAR INFECTIONS?

Very seldom is there only one condition that predisposes a child to otitis media; many factors often combine to cause the ear infections. Some of these factors cannot be controlled by the parent, such as an inherited tendency toward ear infections, the child's age, number of siblings or a poorly functioning eustachian tube. If one of these factors is causing ear troubles in your child, you'll just have to wait until your child "outgrows" the problem since little preventive action can be taken. But other factors *can* be controlled, such as bottle propping and parental smoking. And other factors, such as day care and stress, may lead parents to change their life styles.

One cause of recurrent and persistent otitis media, suggest many experts, is the frequent and/or indiscriminate use of antibiotics in the treatment of otitis media. Some studies have shown that antibiotics create an environment in the middle ear that can cause fluid to linger longer in the ear and perhaps block the body's healing process. These studies are discussed fully in the Antibiotics section.

In general, children who are born with cleft palate and Down syndrome are very likely to suffer middle ear problems. Additionally, many physicians believe children who have allergies are more prone to ear infections than non-allergic children. Children over age four who are still suffering recurrent ear infections are likely to have an underlying cause such as an abnormal palate or allergies.

Even though some factors put children at high risk for ear infections, a great many children who are generally healthy suffer consecutive ear infections and persistent middle ear fluid. Parents may never fully understand the reasons why these children suffer recurrent episodes; but most of these children will "outgrow" their illnesses about age four.

BASIC FACTORS That Cause Otitis Media

Age. Ear infections occur most often in children between the ages of 6 months and 24 months. The incidence of otitis media declines as age increases, except for an upturn when the child enters school.[1]

Sex. Most studies have shown that boys have a greater tendency toward ear infections than girls, although the cause of this has not been determined.[1]

Race. American Indian, Eskimo and Hispanic children have a relatively high number of ear infections. Other studies show that black children have a lower incidence of ear infection than white children.[1]

Inheritance. Children who have recurrent otitis media are likely to have siblings or parents with the same history.[1]

Cleft Palate. A cleft palate is a congenital defect characterized by an opening in roof of the mouth. Otitis media occurs frequently in children under two years of age who have a cleft palate.[2] Even after the palate is repaired, ear infections continue to be a problem. The potential hearing loss from this continual problem can diminish a child's speech and social development.

Children who are born with a cleft palate do not have normal muscles pulling on the eustachian tube. Consequently, their eustachian tubes have difficulty opening and closing, and the tube's "breathing" (or ventilating) function is impaired. Often, even a slight abnormality in a palate can cause recurrent ear infections.

Every child with a cleft palate needs special medical attention and careful evaluation for middle ear problems. Usually, an ENT specialist will recommend insertion of ventilating tubes before the age of six months in a child who has a cleft palate. This assures that the child will not experience hearing loss at an early age and suffer difficulties with speech development beyond the problems associated with a cleft palate.

Down Syndrome. Nearly 60 percent of children with Down syndrome suffer middle ear problems, and the problems continue into adulthood.[3] The muscle that helps control the eustachian tube often does not work well in these children, resulting in poor tube function. Because these children are already at a disadvantage for hearing and language development, many ENT specialists will recommend insertion of ventilating tubes at an early age to avoid persistent middle ear fluid that can cause hearing loss.

BIOLOGIC FACTORS That Cause Otitis Media

Eustachian Tube Dysfunction. The single most frequent factor causing ear infections is poor eustachian tube function resulting in inadequate ventilation of the middle ear.[4] The eustachian tube allows the middle ear to "breathe" as the tube opens and closes with every swallow. A child's eustachian tube can easily become blocked or swollen (called edema). A simple cold can create enough mucus or inflammation to block the eustachian tube. Once the tube becomes blocked, a vacuum is created in the ear because its lining absorbs air and the ear cannot "breathe" in order to replenish the air. Mucus that becomes trapped in the ear, called persistent middle ear fluid, is susceptible to infection.

Bacteria and Viruses are microorganisms that can create inflammation in the tissues of the lining of the middle ear. The most common varieties of bacteria that cause middle ear infection in children are called Hemophilus influenzae and Streptococcus pneumoniae. Another type of bacteria called

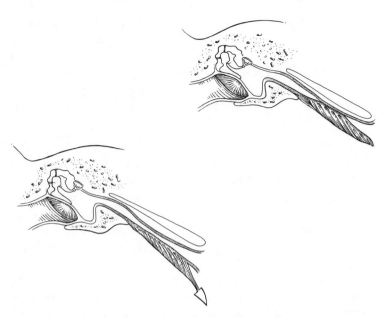

The eustachian tube is closed (top) until muscles are contracted and it opens with a swallow (above).

Branhamella catarrhallis is becoming a relatively common cause of otitis media, especially in young children.[5] Even after a middle ear is no longer acutely infected, bacteria linger in the middle ear fluid of approximately 50 percent of children who have persistent effusion.[6]

Allergy may be a contributing factor in the cause of frequently occurring otitis media and/or persistent middle ear fluid. Inhaled substances—such as house dust, mold spores, grass, tree and weed pollens—are the major offenders responsible for producing symptoms of nasal allergy. Children also may have allergic reactions to certain types of food (especially milk and dairy products). The most frequent sign of allergy is a runny nose. Other signs include: wheezing, sneezing, puffy eyes, headache, itchy nose. Accompanying these signs can be listlessness, moodiness or irritability.

Some allergic children may have severe symptoms during seasons when certain pollen or other plant substances are in the air; the child sensitive to house dust may have worsening symptoms during the cool months of the year when the furnace is on. Musty odors and mold can bring on allergic reactions, as can tobacco smoke.[7] (For discussion of treatment of the allergic child, see page 109.)

Immunity. Our bodies have a natural defense mechanism, called the immune response, to fight against the invasion of infection. Emotional stress that results from unexpected or unhappy events in life—such as a death or divorce in the family—also could lower your child's resistance by causing lack of sleep, fatigue, improper or unbalanced diet and disruption in a child's everyday routine. These, in turn, can interfere with the body's immune mechanism.[8]

A child is susceptible to infection during infancy when the immune system is adjusting to the environment outside the womb. As a child grows older, antibodies develop to fight infection and illness. Children develop antibodies at different rates and in different ways; but most children develop antibodies during upper respiratory infections (colds) and childhood diseases.

Some children's immune systems are unable to produce the defenses needed to fight infection and are more susceptible to disease than are other children. These children are said to have immunodeficiency. Today, researchers are trying to determine why some children seem to develop an ear infection every time they catch a cold or cough. Studies have shown that the local immune mechanism that fights disease in middle ear infections works poorly in some children.[9,10]

Upper Respiratory Infection. Most parents notice that their child develops an ear infection as the acute symptoms of a cold are diminishing. Colds can contribute to swelling of the eustachian tube, which in turn leads to improper functioning. Also, a cold can lead to otitis media if the bacteria or virus causing the cold travels to the middle ear via the eustachian tube.

The common cold also can lead to other upper respiratory infections, such as sinusitis. Sinusitis is inflammation of the lining of the sinuses and can cause pain in and around the sinuses that are inflamed. Both these conditions can predispose a child to ear infections.

Common Childhood Illness. Many childhood illnesses can increase susceptibility to infection because the mucus in the ear can be attacked by the same type of bacteria or virus that causes a childhood disease. Nasal congestion associated with measles, chicken pox, strep throat, whooping cough, scarlet fever and diphtheria increases the chances of an ear infection.[8]

Chronic Illness. Less frequent causes of otitis media could include any chronic illness associated with lowered resistance, such as diabetes or chronic cough.[8]

Abnormal Middle Ear Conditions. Recurrent middle ear infections can damage cilia, which are short, hairlike extensions of cells that help to move mucus out of the middle ear and through the eustachian tube. Infections can also alter the chemical properties of the mucus, making it a thick, gluelike fluid that is more likely to persist for longer periods of time.[11]

Adenoids. During normal development, a child's adenoids may become unusually large. Some researchers believe that enlarged adenoids can push against the eustachian tube and interfere with ventilation.[3] (See discussion of adenoidectomy in Part Three.)

ENVIRONMENTAL FACTORS That Cause Otitis Media

Bottle Propping means lying a child on his back in bed and propping the bottle in his mouth for long periods of time. This age-old practice seems innocuous enough, but some researchers have found it to be a leading factor in the development of

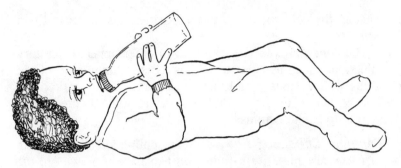

One major preventative measure that parents can take is to NEVER put their children to bed or lay their children down with a bottle. The fluid can be sucked up into the eustachian tube, carrying dangerous bacteria to the middle ear.

persistent middle ear fluid in infants and toddlers.[12] As the milk flows out of the bottle into a reclining child's mouth, fluid (and its accompanying bacteria) can be sucked up into the eustachian tube.

Cigarette Smoke. Otitis media has been shown to occur more frequently in children who live with smokers.[11,13,14] Cigarette smoke can irritate the mucus membranes lining the nasal and middle ear cavities, causing dysfunction of the eustachian tube.

Day Care. Children experience many colds and other illnesses during the first five years of life. If exposed to other children on a daily basis, the chances increase that a child will develop more illnesses. Many researchers studying the origin of middle ear disease say the increasing use of day care centers has led to a rise in the number of cases of otitis media. A recent study, comparing children who stayed at home with children in day care, showed that those in day care suffered more persistent middle ear fluid, and in most cases poorer hearing, than the children who were cared for at home. The researchers concluded this was attributable to the increased risk of contamination of the children in day care.[15,16]

Climate. Damp, humid climates can contribute to a child's chances for infections. Children tend to develop ear infections during the winter months when upper respiratory infections occur frequently. Highest monthly rates of ear infections occur in January through March with the lowest rates in July and August. For children with pollen or plant-substance allergies, the spring season may contribute to an increase in ear infections.[1]

Socioeconomic. Any of the factors that contribute to poverty can contribute to a higher incidence of ear infections: overcrowded living conditions; damp, chilly housing; malnutrition; unhygienic personal habits; poor sanitation; polluted environments; infrequent or inadequate medical care.[1]

Sniffing/Blowing the Nose. Some researchers have been studying whether these two practices can contribute to ear infection. Some researchers claim that sniffing clears all air from the middle ear, causing negative pressure.[17] Similarly, other researchers claim that blowing the nose also causes the spread of bacteria and viruses into the middle ear as the mucus travels up the nasopharynx and gets trapped in the eustachian tube.[18]

QUESTIONS AND ANSWERS ════

Q: Are ear infections contagious?

A: No, but an upper respiratory infection (common cold) that often precedes an ear infection is contagious.

Q: If a child is prone to ear infections, are there special precautions that must be taken on a plane trip?

A: Rapid changes in air pressure can occur as a plane descends (especially in small planes with cabins that are not as pressurized as large planes). In order to avoid that "blocked-

up" feeling, the eustachian tube must open frequently while the plane is going from low atmospheric pressure at high altitudes to the high pressure closer to earth. These pressure changes can also be experienced on a smaller scale in an elevator or when diving to the bottom of a swimming pool.

You may have noticed that, as a plane is landing, the babies on the plane tend to cry or fuss. Infants are especially susceptible to these pressure changes and may be in great ear pain during descent and afterwards.

A child, whether or not he is prone to ear infections, should be kept awake during ascent and descent of the plane. Infants can suck on bottle, breast or pacifier; older children can chew gum, yawn or suck on a hard candy or food. Although not guaranteed to prevent ear infections, it may be worthwhile to give your child both orally administered decongestant medication and also nasal spray decongestant one half hour before descent to help shrink the membranes and possibly help the eustachian tube function more effectively.

Q: At what point should I consult an allergist if I suspect my child is allergic to food or environment?

A: Probably not until your child is more than four years old. Since ear infections are so common in early childhood, it's unnecessary to evaluate for allergies every child who has frequent ear infections. After age four, however, ear infections usually decrease in an otherwise healthy child. If not, evaluation for allergy may be worthwhile, especially if your child suffers from a frequent runny nose and sneezing and has dark circles beneath the eyes, itchy skin, rashes or eczema. Another reason to wait until age four is that the older child is better able to cooperate for allergy skin tests and for any medical therapy that may be advised for treatment of the allergies.

Q: Are children more prone to get ear infections when they're teething?

A: Many parents incorrectly think a relationship exists between teething and ear infections because they seem to occur simultaneously. Both teething and ear infections are a common occurrence during childhood, but there is no evidence to show that teething in any way causes ear infections.

Q: If a child doesn't wear a hat in cold or windy weather, can he get an ear infection?

A: There is no relationship between cold or windy weather and ear infections. The best action for parents to take is to use common sense in dressing their children for extremes in weather.

RESEARCH

Who is the "otitis-prone" child and what factors contribute to this condition? The answer to this question has a high priority for experts exploring the causes of otitis media. Researchers are conducting studies on infectious, genetic, environmental and nutritional factors that can possibly predispose a child to otitis media. Three areas in which research is being conducted include:

Allergy: Some studies indicate that allergy may play a significant role in otitis media's development; others question this finding. Experts are calling for more extensive studies on this subject.[1,18]

Eustachian Tube. Animals have been used extensively in the study of the anatomy and the function of the eustachian tube. But researchers claim that "the most fundamental physiologic information (about the eustachian tube) is still lacking and the number of researchers who are active in this field is diminishing.''[19] Information about the anatomy of the eustachian tube is considered essential to understanding how the eustachian tube contributes to otitis media.[20]

Immune Response. Researchers at the Children's Hospital of Pittsburgh are studying how the immune mechanism works in the middle ear and its possible role in causing and prolonging ear infections.[21]

NOTES ▬▬▬▬▬▬▬▬▬▬▬▬▬▬▬▬▬▬

1. Giebink GS. "Epidemiology and Natural History of Otitis Media" in Recent Advances in Otitis Media with Effusion. (DJ Lim, Editor in Chief). BC Decker Inc., 1984: 5–9.

2. Paradise JL. "Otitis Media in Infants and Children." Pediatrics 1980 May; 65 (5): 920.

3. Curtis AW, Clemis JD. "Middle Ear Effusions: Part 1—Pathophysiology." The Journal of Continuing Education in O.R.L. and Allergy. 1979 May: 13-25.

4. Cantekin EI. "State of the Art: Physiology and Pathophysiology of the Eustatchian Tube" in Recent Advances in Otitis Media With Effusion (DJ Lim, Editor in Chief), BC Decker Inc., 1984: 45–52.

5. Nelson JD. "State of the Art: Microbiology of Acute Otitis Media With Effusion" in Recent Advances in Otitis Media With Effusion (DJ Lim, Editor in Chief), BC Decker Inc., 1984: 105–106.

6. Lim DJ, DeMaria TF. "Bacteriology and Immunology." Laryngoscope. 1982 March: 92 (3): 278–286.

7. Miller DL, Friday GA. Allergic Diseases of the Nose and Middle Ear in Children. Ear, Nose and Throat Journal. 1978 March; 57; 27–115.

8. Proctor B. "Etiology of Otitis Media" in Otitis Media, publication of the Second National Conference on Otitis Media (coeditors RJ Weit, SW Coulthard) 1979 January; Ross Laboratories, Columbus, Ohio: 21–25.

9. Bluestone CD, Klein JO. "Otitis Media with Effusion, Atelectasis and Eustachian Tube Dysfunction" in Pediatric Otolaryngology Volume 1 (edited by CD Bluestone and SE Stool). 1983 WB Saunders Co.: 410.

10. Ogra PL, Chairman. "Microbiology, Immunology, Biochemistry and Vaccination" in Recent Advances in Otitis Media With Effusion (DJ Lim, Editor). Annals of Otol, Rhinol, Laryngol. 1985 Jan–Feb; Suppl 116: 94 (1)(3): 18-22.

11. Kraemer MJ; Richardson MA, et al. "Risk Factors for Persistent Middle Ear Effusion. Otitis Media, catarrh, cigarette smoke exposure and atopy." JAMA. 1983 Feb. 25; 249 (8): 1022–25.

12. Teele DW, Klein JO, Rosner B. Epidemiology of Otitis Media in Children. Ann Otol Rhinol Laryngol May–June 1980; 89 (suppl 68): 5–6.

13. Pukander J, Luotonen J, Timonen M, Karma P. Risk Factors Affecting the Occurrence of Acute Otitis Media Among 2-3-Year-Old Urban Children. Acta Otolaryngol (Stockh) 1985 Sep–Oct; 100 (3–4): 260–265.

14. Black, Nick. The Aetiology of Glue Ear — A Case-Control Study. Int J of Pediatric Otorhinolaryngology. 1985 Jul: 9(2): 121–133.

15. B Vinther, B Pedersen, Elbrond O. "Otitis Media in Childhood. Sociomedical Aspects with Special Reference to Day-Care Situations." Clin Otolaryngol. 1984 Feb: 9 (1): 3–8.

16. B Vinther, Elbrond O. "A Population Study of Otitis Media in Childhood." Acto Otolaryngol (Stockh) Suppl 360:135, 1979.

17. Magnuson B, Falk B. "New Techniques for Measuring Eustachian Tube Responses" in Recent Advances in Otitis Media With Effusion (DJ Lim, Editor in Chief); BC Decker Inc, 1984: 49–52.

18. Bluestone CD, Klein JO. "Otitis Media with Effusion, Atelectasis and Eustachian Tube Dysfunction" in Pediatric Otolaryngology Volume 1 (edited by CD Bluestone and SE Stool). 1983 WB Saunders Co.: 398.

19. Cantekin EI. "Eustachian Tube and Middle Ear Physiology and Pathophysiology" in Recent Advances in Otitis Media With Effusion (DJ Lim, editor). Ann Otol, Rhin & Laryngol. 1985 Jan–Feb. Suppl 116:94(Part 1, No. 3):12–13.

20. Lim DJ, Chairman. "Anatomy, Cell Biology and Pathology" in Recent Advances in Otitis Media With Effusion (DJ Lim, editor). Ann Otol, Rhin & Laryngol. 1985 Jan–Feb. Suppl 116:94(Part 1, No. 3):14–17.

21. Information based on list of CRISP records of currently active USPHS grants and contracts and NIH intramural projects active in 1988 from the Division of Research Grants, Department of Health and Human Services, Public Health Service.

CHAPTER FOUR

Diagnosis and Examination

What Causes the Ache in an Earache?

The term earache is often used when describing the pain that accompanies an ear infection. An earache can be a dull, throbbing pain that robs the child of spark and energy and renders him listless and abnormally quiet; the earache can be so sharp that the child screams out and writhes in pain; or the earache can simply be a nagging discomfort that makes the child tug at his ear or rub his face in an attempt to ease the pain.

Ear pain is caused when infected fluid accumulates in the middle ear and exerts pressure against the eardrum. As the fluid increases in volume, it pushes more and more against the pliable eardrum, stretching it to its breaking point. At this point, the condition is considered acute, and can cause one or all of the following symptoms: fever, lethargy, irritability, crying, sleeplessness, restlessness, drainage from the ear.

Some children will show no symptoms of ear pain until the eardrum is about to burst; often children awaken in the middle of the night, feverish and screaming in pain. Other children exhibit telltale signs as soon as the fluid begins to collect in the middle ear because the infection is affecting their overall health, causing low-grade fever, loss of appetite, tiredness or irritability.

Severe ear pain can develop quickly and dramatically; a child who was content and happy at bedtime can awaken five hours later screaming in agony. One mother remembers an incident when her child's ears were pronounced healthy during a routine checkup and, the next day, the child was back in the doctor's office suffering acute otitis media.

Sometimes, the body's defense system may prevent the infected fluid from accumulating to the point where it presses against the eardrum. If this occurs, many parents won't even know their child has an ear infection. Even if they suspect that an ear infection is developing, they may wait a few days to see if the infection "runs its course" before taking the child to the doctor.

Every Child Has Unique Symptoms

Each child's symptoms of ear discomfort are unique and may vary from one infection to another, depending on its severity. Most parents use a combination of intuition, experience and education to determine if a child is suffering ear pain. After a child has had several ear infections, parents may detect a pattern of symptoms or behavior that signals the child is experiencing ear pain. Perhaps the child acts different or is "not himself." As one mother said, "Adam never ran a fever, but when he started having a runny nose, we'd worry. If he had watery-looking eyes, it almost always meant he had an ear infection."

Another mother recognized her son's way of showing he had an ear infection: he would tug on his ears and rub the side of his face.

Although ear infections are classically linked with symptoms of fever and ear pain, parents should note that *fever and/ or ear pain does not automatically indicate an ear infection.*[1] One group of physicians found that 30% of patients in a survey did not have an ear infection even though the parents said the child complained of an earache. Many of these children had colds or viral illnesses.[1A] Likewise, a child's habit of tugging

Symptoms of Ear Infections

- Fever
- Crying
- Restlessness
- Inability to sleep
- Lethargy
- Glassy eyes
- Loss of appetite
- Not wanting to suck on pacifier, bottle or breast
- Irritability
- Whining, clinging to parent
- Tugging at ear
- Rubbing side of face
- Drainage from ear

at the ears does not mean the child has an ear infection. This "symptom" can merely be a habit or comfort gesture for many children, much like thumb sucking. For instance, some children will automatically start tugging at their ears when they're hungry, tired, or when they feel discomfort from teething.

Signs of Persistent Middle Ear Fluid

Fluid in the ear can persist for weeks, or even months, without any symptoms whatsoever. Many children adjust to the "plugged-up" feeling of middle ear fluid and carry on with no complaint.

However, other children feel a nagging discomfort when

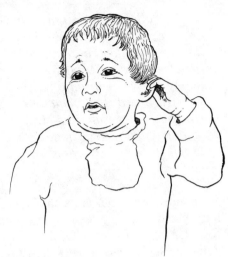

Many infants and toddlers tug at their ears when they have an ear infection. But tugging at the ears does not necessarily mean the child has an ear infection. This habit can be compared to sucking the thumb—some children do it often as a comfort gesture to mean they are hungry or tired.

fluid persists in the middle ear. This discomfort can be complicated by hearing loss that can accompany persistent effusion (see Part Six for a complete explanation). Your child also may awaken at night if he feels the movement of fluid from side to side as he turns in his sleep. Other symptoms may include pulling at the ear and irritability.

Physicians routinely examine children's ears during well-baby and well-child visits, and often detect fluid in the middle ear. Unless this fluid has persisted for more than three months, or is causing hearing loss or ear pain, you and your doctor will probably decide to withhold treatment and give the fluid a chance to subside spontaneously.

WHEN IS IT TIME TO VISIT THE DOCTOR? ▬

Is It an Earache or a New Tooth?

One of the most frustrating tasks of a new parent is determining if an infant is sick, or if he's just having a grouchy day.

"We always wondered if it would be better to just observe the baby at home for a couple of days and let the ear infection run its course," said one mother. "I preferred that to bringing him to the pediatrician and letting him wait in an office with other sick children. I was frustrated that I couldn't just look in his ears and see if they were infected. Even after I got all the information about recognizing ear infections, it was still hard to tell if an ear infection was the cause of irritable behavior."

Parents of infants are usually unsure about what "symptoms" can mean. Is teething the cause of the baby's discomfort? Or is she hungry? Or does she have a stomachache? Or could these symptoms be a sign that she is developing acute otitis media?

The parent of a toddler or preschooler can question the child about his discomfort. Even at that age, however, children sometimes are unable to identify where they hurt. They know they're uncomfortable, but they're not sure if it's their stomach or ear, or if they're just tired or hungry. As the child gets older, signs of illness become more recognizable and eventually he can tell you whether or not he's sick. But there's still the same dilemma: when is a child sick enough to be taken to the doctor?

Parents who don't take their child to a doctor may fear they're ignoring a serious problem, and parents who take their child to the doctor at the first suspicion of an ear infection may worry that they will be labelled as alarmists.

A fever higher than 102 degrees Fahrenheit or apparent unremitting ear pain could indicate the ear infection is quite severe, or there may be another cause for the symptoms. Therefore, if your child has a very high fever or seems inconsolable, then bring your child to a physician promptly.

In many cases, however, a parent could postpone a trip to the physician for 24 hours to give the ear infection and its accompanying symptoms a chance to clear up. [*Ed. note:*

When Is It Time to Visit the Doctor?

Acute otitis media:

Symptoms of ear pain, such as crying, fever, lethargy for more than 24 hours

Follow-Up

If acute symptoms do not subside despite antimicrobial treatment, return to physician.
If hearing loss is suspected, return to physician.

Several studies show that 70 to 80 percent of untreated cases of acute otitis media will resolve within 24 to 72 hours.[2,3,4]
If the child is exhibiting acute symptoms of pain, ease the child's discomfort by applying a warm towel or washcloth to the sore ear and giving him a non-aspirin liquid or tablet pain reliever. If after 24 hours the acute symptoms still persist, the child should be seen by a physician.

What about the 20 to 30 percent of children whose ear infections do *not* resolve spontaneously? If the parents take the child to the doctor at the first sign of ear pain, could antimicrobial treatment prevent the fluid from building up to the point where it causes severe ear pain? Although it is logical to assume that early treatment with an antibiotic might prevent later build-up of fluid in the middle ear, there really is no scientific evidence to show that every child needs immediate antibiotic treatment for every ear infection.

Determining when to bring your child to a doctor for treatment of an ear infection largely depends upon how you view the role of a physician in providing health care. Many parents feel obligated to check out any symptom that may indicate an ear infection is present and are willing to put their child on antimicrobial treatment ''just in case'' an ear infection occurs.

Others are content to take the chance that the infection will resolve without treatment. As one mother put it, her child had been put on antibiotics so many times that it was like "taking an aspirin for a headache that you never get." A more complete discussion of these two views is presented in Part Four.

DIAGNOSIS

The eardrum is like a window to the inside of the middle ear. The experienced eye of a physician can see if fluid is bulging against the window, trying to escape; or he can see bubbles that are trapped behind the window, indicating fluid is in the middle ear; or he can see a healthy window that is translucent with a shiny gray color. To a parent, however, the ear examination may be confusing because the physician is examining something hidden and invisible. Many parents have no concept of what the physician sees or what he is looking for when he looks through the examining instrument, and very few question the physician's diagnosis.

For parents to take an active role in management of their children's ear infections, they should have a basic understanding of how a physician examines the ear.

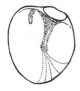

On the left is a healthy eardrum as viewed through an otoscope. The physician can see the "landmarks" of the eardrum, that is, he can see the protrusion of certain bones. In the right drawing, the eardrum is bulging and inflamed and the physician can no longer see any landmarks.

PURPOSES OF EXAMINATIONS ▬▬▬▬

The Examination: Acute Otitis Media

The physician examines the child who has an earache to confirm the presence of fluid. An ear examination under these circumstances can be a distressing experience, because the child cringes when his ear is touched, and parents are upset about the child's reactions. Most likely, your child will cry and struggle to get away from the physician. Though it may be impossible for you to calm your child during the examination, it's essential for you to stay relaxed and help the child remain still and cooperative.

Why is it necessary for the physician to examine an unhappy, struggling child if the child's symptoms obviously point to an ear infection? Couldn't this uncomfortable examination be avoided? Couldn't the physician simply prescribe antibiotics without looking at the ear?

No matter how unpleasant the ear examination can be for parents, child and physician, a doctor must see the eardrum to diagnose otitis media. The child could have another illness that causes symptoms similar to those of an ear infection, or the ear may need more serious and immediate treatment. Most physicians do not condone the practice of prescribing antibiotics for an ear infection unless that diagnosis has been made after an examination. Although some physicians may tell parents that a child has an ear infection after merely listening to a description of symptoms, this practice can lead to inaccurate diagnosis and inappropriate or excessive treatment.

The Examination: Well-Baby Visit

Pediatricians routinely examine the ears during well-baby visits to check for fluid in the middle ear that is not causing symptoms. If a pediatrician sees middle ear fluid during a well-baby visit, the parent and physician may want to discuss whether treatment is necessary, or whether a hearing test is appropriate to determine hearing loss (see Part Six). If the pediatrician diagnoses acute otitis media in a presumably healthy child during a well-baby visit, the parent may question what led him to that conclusion and why the child is not showing any symptoms of pain.

The Examination: The ENT Specialist

Your child probably may be referred to an otolaryngologist, commonly known as an Ear, Nose and Throat (ENT) specialist, because he is suffering frequently occurring otitis media (more than four episodes in each of two consecutive seasons) or persistent middle ear effusion (fluid in one or both ears for more than 10 weeks).

The ENT specialist will examine not only your child's ears, but also his nose and throat. He will examine the child's nose

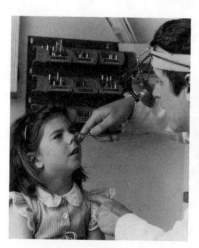 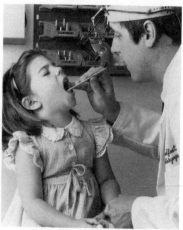

A complete examination by an ENT specialist includes a search for underlying causes of otitis media, such as allergy or abnormal palate. The physician not only examines the ear, but the throat and nose as well. *(Photos by Donna K. Cantor)*

for signs of allergy, such as swelling, or for signs of chronic infection. The throat is examined for infection, or to see if the palate is normally shaped. The specialist will feel behind the ears for tenderness that could mean mastoiditis, and he will look for any skin condition that could be associated with allergies. Finally, he will listen to the child's speech and voice quality.

DIFFICULTIES IN EXAMINATION

A squirming, uncooperative child and/or an ear full of wax complicate ear examinations for any physician, no matter how many thousands of ears he has looked at. It's crucial for the physician to be able to thoroughly view the eardrum and to see how the eardrum moves when air pressure is applied with a rubber bulb.

This difficult job is made harder by two additional factors:

Shape of ear canal. Every child's ear canal is shaped differently, and every eardrum looks different. Some children's ear canals may be very narrow or twisted, making it particularly difficult to view the middle ear.

Flexibility of ear canal. The compliance of the external ear canal changes as the child grows older. In the newborn, the ear canal is so flexible that a physician can have trouble seeing through to the eardrum. Some physicians may think they are seeing the eardrum move back and forth, when, in fact, they are viewing the ear canal. The experienced physician will admit that some children have eardrums that are difficult to examine. In infants under six weeks of age it is extraordinarily difficult to diagnose an ear infection through a routine ear examination. Quite often, diagnosis of ear infection in young babies is so difficult the doctor may put a needle through the eardrum just to determine the presence of middle ear fluid.

Restraining the Child

To keep an infant's head still, the doctor may ask you to lay the infant down on the examining table while you hold his head. If the child is a toddler, it may be easier to sit the child in your lap, wrapping your arms around his torso and head. The physician may call in an assistant to help you restrain the uncooperative toddler or preschooler. If the child cannot be kept still by the parent and assistant, he may have to be restrained in a "papoose"—a board fitted with a series of paired Velcro® straps that immobilizes the child's limbs. Very few children tolerate this experience without immediately beginning to cry.

Ways That Physician Removes Wax from Ear

1) Flushing ear canal with water
2) Aspiration
3) Manual removal with curette

Removing Earwax

Before the physician can clearly see the eardrum, he must remove any earwax (called cerumen) that is blocking his view of the ear canal. (Note: a parent should never use cotton tipped swabs to remove wax from a child's ear. With one quick turn of the child's head, you may puncture the eardrum.) There are several ways a physician removes wax from the canal:

Flushing the ear canal with water. This can be done with a special ear cleansing syringe or with an electronic water pump.

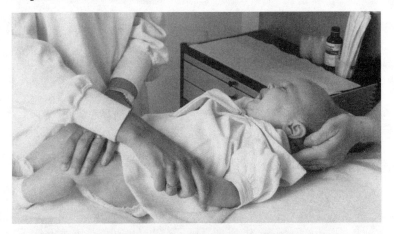

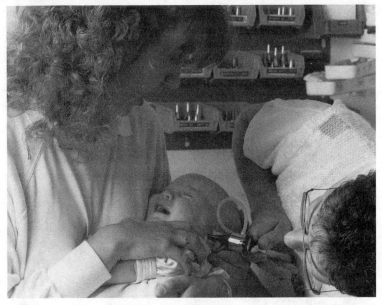

An infant can be examined in two ways: either by lying the child on an examining table, with the parent and assistant holding the legs, arms and head; or by the parent holding the child close to her chest with her hands restraining the head. *(Photos by Donna K. Cantor)*

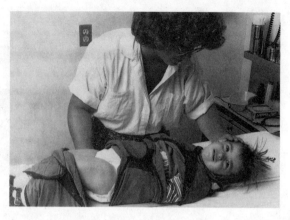

A squirming, uncooperative child should never be an excuse for a physician to conduct an incomplete ear examination. If necessary, the child can be restrained by a "papoose," as shown above. Two adults can help restrain the child by holding her head while the doctor examines the ears. Although the child may be frightened and feel uncomfortable because of the restraint, many parents prefer a short amount of discomfort in return for a thorough examination and an accurate diagnosis. *(Photo by Donna K. Cantor)*

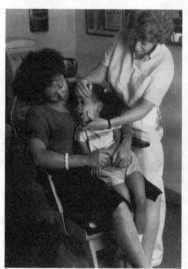

An older child can be restrained by the parent wrapping the legs around the child's legs, wrapping one arm around the child's chest and holding the head back. An uncooperative child can be held in the same manner with the assistance of a second adult. *(Photo by Donna K. Cantor)*

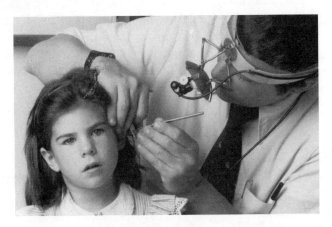

Before a physician can visualize the eardrum, the ear canal must be clear of wax. Above, a physician has inserted a speculum into the child's ear and uses a curette to remove the wax. Other means of removing ear wax include flushing the ear canal with water and gentle suction with an aspirator. *(Photo by Donna K. Cantor)*

Gentle suction with an aspirator permits removal of material not only from the ear canal, but from the surface of the eardrum itself.

Manual removal with a curette. The doctor may manually remove the wax from the ear canal by using a curette, a long, thin instrument with a smooth, rounded head. To best manipulate the curette, the doctor may insert a funnel shaped instrument called a speculum into the outer ear.

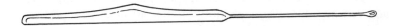

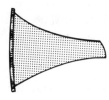

One way in which physicians clean out wax in the ear is with a curette (top) and speculum. The narrow portion of the speculum is inserted into the ear and allows the physician better visualization of the wax and better control as he is removing the wax with the rounded tip of the curette.

At times, cleaning of the ear canal can lead to bleeding. This is caused when an instrument tears or scrapes the skin of the ear canal. This bleeding is usually slight and does not interfere with observation of the eardrum or cause any health hazard.

WHAT THE PHYSICIAN SEES DURING EXAMINATION

The Physician's Instruments

The kind of magnifying instrument a physician uses to view the eardrum is crucial to the accuracy of diagnosis. The best ear-examining instrument, a pneumatic otoscope, is usually made of chromed steel or plastic and has a halogen bulb to illuminate the ear canal to allow viewing of all parts of the eardrum.

The pneumatic otoscope fits into the ear and seals the ear canal. The physician can force air into the ear canal to test the mobility of the eardrum by gently blowing into the canal through a tube attached to the otoscope, or by squeezing air into the canal with the instrument's rubber bulb. Squeezing the bulb produces a positive pressure; releasing the bulb creates a negative pressure. This procedure would cause a healthy eardrum to move back and forth, while fluid in the middle ear would interfere with its normal movement.

Even with the pneumatic otoscope, diagnosis is subjective and can be imprecise depending on the physician's expertise; without the otoscope, diagnosis is far more variable and less accurate. At the Otitis Media Research Center in Pittsburgh, researchers must be "validated" in the use of the otoscope so test results will be valid. In other words, a physician's diagnosis must correspond with that of two out of three more experienced examiners.

Some otolaryngologists may view the eardrum with an

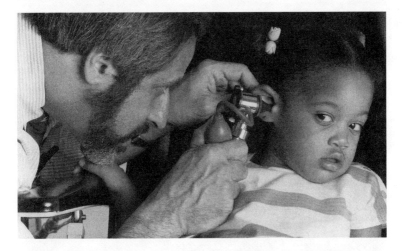

Diagnosis of otitis media is best determined by use of a pneumatic otoscope. Above, the physician squeezes the bulb attached to the otoscope, which gently presses air into the ear canal to test the compliancy of the eardrum. *(Photo by Donna K. Cantor)*

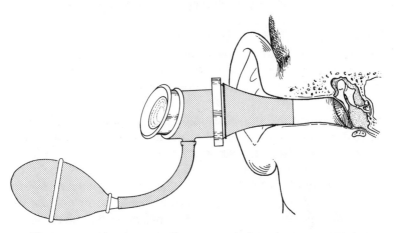

The pneumatic otoscope fits so snugly into the ear canal that it "seals" the ear canal. Therefore, when the physician squeezes the bulb, he gently pumps air in and out of the canal, which causes a healthy eardrum to move back and forth.

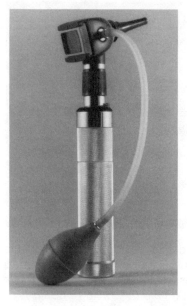

The pneumatic otoscope.
(Photo by Jerry A. McCoy)

otomicroscope. Many otolaryngologists and some pediatricians also use the tympanometer, which can help detect presence of fluid in the middle ear. The tympanometer tests the flexibility of the eardrum by sending a tone down the ear canal, and measuring how much of that tone is absorbed by the eardrum (see Part Six for thorough discussion of tympanometry).

A new instrument now available to physicians is called the acoustic otoscope and detects middle ear fluid by reflecting sound waves off the eardrum. The method, called acoustic reflectometry, has two important benefits: a seal to test mobility of the eardrum need not be created; and the method is reliable regardless of a patient's age, crying, presence of earwax or lack of cooperation. Cost, too, is a consideration: the acoustic otoscope, small enough to fit into a pocket, costs approximately $900,[5,6] while a tympanometer costs at least double.

A study at the Hospital of the University of Pennsylvania also found the acoustic otoscope helpful in identifying middle ear fluid in newborns in the hospital's intensive care unit;

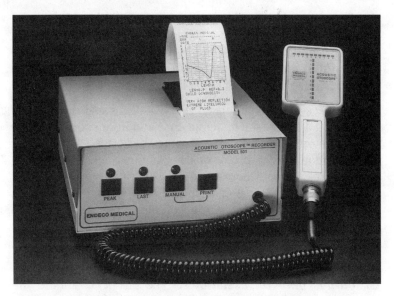

The acoustic otoscope is a handheld instrument that detects middle ear effusion by reflecting sound waves off the eardrum. *(Photo courtesy of Endeco Medical Inc.)*

typically, visual inspection of infants' eardrums is difficult because of small or compliant canals.[7]

What Makes a Good Ear Examiner?

How a physician examines a child can give a parent important clues about the physician's overall approach to the treatment of otitis media. If parents are confident the physician has given their child a thorough examination, they will be comfortable with the resultant diagnosis and suggestions for treatment. Conversely, parents may be less willing to accept a physician's diagnosis if they suspect he has given their child a token or cursory examination (See Part Seven for comprehensive discussion of the physician's role in examination.)

How can a parent evaluate a physician's examination? Below are characteristics parents should look for in determining the thoroughness of the doctor's examination:

Gentle approach. The doctor should approach the child gently, engaging him or her in conversation; in general, he should make the child feel comfortable. The doctor also should be respectful to both parent and child, and avoid "baby talk," a condescending attitude or a harsh approach.

Avoid force. An experienced physician is capable of gently examining a child even under adverse conditions, or will know when to stop when the child becomes hysterical. One mother says her daughter's dislike of ear examinations started when a pediatrician "held her down and stuck the otoscope in her ear so violently that he caused bleeding." Even if a child is struggling and crying, this kind of force is unnecessary and intolerable. If the child is too hysterical for a safe examination, the physician and parent may decide to postpone the visit for several days.

Encourage parental assistance. The physician should instruct the parent how to hold the child's head during the examination. A child may be more comfortable and cooperative if the parent is a part of the examination; likewise, a parent may feel more useful if he or she is able to assist.

Use proper instruments. A good ear examiner will use the proper examining instruments; a pneumatic otoscope is best for observing movement of the eardrum. To further assess the status of the middle ear, the physician can use additional instruments such as an acoustic otoscope or tympanometer.

View eardrum. Since good visualization of the eardrum is painstaking, the good physician will spend whatever time necessary to examine the eardrum to assess mobility and observe landmarks.

Remove wax. If earwax obstructs the physician's view of the eardrum, the wax must be carefully removed.

Summarize findings. After examination and diagnosis, a physician should record in the child's medical record a summary of important findings, including a picture of the child's eardrum so the doctor can accurately recall the eardrum appearance at the follow-up visit. A one word diagnosis or abbreviation, such as "ear infection," "SOM" (serous otitis media) or "AOM" (acute otitis media) is not as helpful as a concise description of relevant symptoms, the course of treatment and abnormal physical findings.

Describe condition to parents. When discussing the diagnosis with parents, the physician should use simple but meaningful terms such as redness, bulging, or dullness of the eardrum. A physician who says your child's eardrum "doesn't look too bad" or "looks junky to me" is doing you a disservice because he's not telling you anything of real substance. Make sure you understand what your doctor is saying even if the physician has to repeat himself.

Color, Landmarks, Mobility

Once the child has been restrained and wax has been removed from the ear, the physician looks for three clues to determine if an ear infection is present:

Color and reflective quality of the eardrum. The eardrum normally appears brilliantly translucent under the light of a physician's otoscope. With acute otitis media, the eardrum loses its luster and may appear yellow, with a pink or red hue, or even dull gray.

What the Physician Looks for Through the Otoscope

1) Color of eardrum
2) Bones that provide "landmarks" to the physician
3) Mobility of the eardrum
4) Bubbles in the middle ear that denote fluid

To some doctors, the absence of a "light reflex" means a child has an ear infection because an infected eardrum loses the normal shiny surface that brilliantly reflects the otoscope's light. Actually, this is a most unreliable indicator of middle ear infection and is not valid as the sole determinant for diagnosis. A child with a severe ear infection can have a normal light reflex and a child with normal eardrums may have a poor light reflex. In general, doctors who have not learned well the telltale signs of ear infection will concentrate on and speak about the light reflex.

Visibility of certain "landmarks." Certain bones visible through the eardrum provide "landmarks" to the physician. If these landmarks cannot be seen, the physician assumes the eardrum is bulging, or it has become opaque to such an extent as to obscure a view of the bones.

Mobility of the eardrum. It is especially important for the physician to test if the eardrum can move back and forth. If the ear is full of fluid, the eardrum does not move back and forth briskly as the examiner exerts air pressure on the eardrum with the bulb on the pneumatic otoscope.

After your doctor has examined your child's ears, ask him what signs he has observed that led to his diagnosis. If your child is cooperative, the physician may also let you observe the eardrum through the otoscope.

OVERDIAGNOSING AND MISDIAGNOSING ▄▄▄▄

The difficult task of examining children's ears can lead, in many instances, to misdiagnosis or overdiagnosis of otitis media. Most often, a physician errs on the "safe" side—that is, he prescribes medication even when he's unsure about the presence of ear infection.

"I became suspicious of the constant antibiotics that my doctor was prescribing for my daughter," said one parent. "Then when an ENT specialist examined my daughter's ears,

How Parent Can Take an Active Role in the Examination

Ask questions

Expect respect from physician

Comfort and calm child

Ask physician to be specific when describing condition and explaining diagnosis

Has the physician seen the eardrum? What did it look like?

Schedule another time for conference if child is crying

he said it was not an acute infection, just persistent effusion, and antimicrobial treatment wasn't really necessary.'' A parent's instinct against excessive use of antibiotics may be correct; many experts now theorize overmedication may be a factor in the prevalence of chronic ear problems.

Less often does a physician underestimate an ear

Causes of Overdiagnoses, Misdiagnoses

Physician assumes red eardrum means infection

Physician can't see eardrum because of wax or because child is struggling

Hurried, incomplete examination

Physician assumes fluid means infection

Parents may influence physician to prescribe antibiotics

condition— but it does happen. In one instance, when a nine-year-old boy was referred to an ENT specialist for a possible cholesteatoma (a harmful substance that builds up behind the eardrum), the specialist found a tube implanted in his eardrum that had become infected by debris. Neither a pediatrician nor another specialist had spotted the tube; in fact, they said the tube had dropped out months earlier. By the time the boy was examined by the second ENT specialist, the skin that began growing around the tube had become infected. The specialist prescribed ear drops to clear up the infection and reduce swelling of infected areas on the eardrum; a week later, he removed the tube.

A physician can overdiagnose or misdiagnose otitis media in the following ways:

Assuming a red eardrum is a sign of an infection. When children cry, their eardrums often become engorged with blood, leading to a red eardrum. Although a red eardrum does accompany many cases of otitis media, it should not be the sole basis for diagnosis. In fact, an infected eardrum is more likely to appear yellow than red.

Not looking for anatomical landmarks. A study at the Bowman Gray School of Medicine at Wake Forest University in Winston-Salem, N.C., was conducted to determine if pediatric residents (physicians who are learning to become pediatricians) could identify the top of the eardrum (the pars flacida), an area which usually bulges first in an ear infection.[8] More than half—53 percent—were unable to identify the pars flacida either on paper or by direct observation through an otoscope.

"Most of the pediatric residents argued they didn't need to know the anatomy to diagnose otitis media," says Ronald B. Mack, M.D., associate professor of pediatrics, who conducted the study. "We have a feeling many pediatricians . . . diagnose otitis media on the basis of whether an eardrum is red, and that doesn't mean anything by itself because if the baby cries, the eardrum gets red; you can't make the diagnosis solely on color of the eardrum."

The study led Dr. Mack to conclude that residents must spend more time studying eardrum anatomy because of its importance in diagnosis.

"We have to be more diligent in emphasizing the anatomy because this is the most common thing that a pediatrician is going to see in his or her practice," he says.

Some physicians believe an ear infection melts earwax. So, if they see earwax, they assume the child does not have an ear infection. However, the presence of earwax does not mean an ear is not infected; nor does the presence of liquified earwax mean an ear *is* infected.[9] A proper diagnosis cannot be made if wax is blocking the ear canal, because it prevents a proper look at the eardrum. One mother said a pediatrician prescribed an antibiotic for her son after telling her there was a "glob of wax" obstructing his view of the eardrum. The mother took the child to another doctor, who thoroughly cleaned the ear canal and saw no signs of otitis media.

Cursory or token examination. A physician may "give up" examining a child because the child's ear canal is too narrow, or because the child is struggling. Some physicians, even if they haven't observed the eardrum, will attribute an infant's fussiness and fever to an ear infection and will subsequently prescribe an antibiotic. This approach is not condoned by most physicians, who believe a firm, factual diagnosis must be established before treatment is given.

Assuming fluid means infection. Many doctors equate the presence of middle ear fluid with an ear infection. However, if the eardrum is not inflamed and bulging, and the child is not complaining of ear pain, then the child does not have acute otitis media. The fluid may be the residual of an ear infection, and most probably will subside without medication within 1 to 3 months. If the fluid does not subside within 3 months, or the child complains of hearing loss, a doctor may prescribe a trial course of antibiotics to clear up the fluid.

A distraught parent may influence the physician to prescribe antibiotics, even though the physician is unsure of the diagnosis or would not ordinarily prescribe medication for the child's condition. Some parents seem reluctant to leave a doctor's office without a prescription; in fact, doctors have remarked that patients complain they're ''not getting their money's worth'' unless the doctor prescribes medication.

Assuming ear infection. If a doctor can't find the cause of a child's fever, he may become frustrated and seek a plausible explanation. Since middle ear fluid can often be observed even in healthy children, a doctor may be tempted to label it as the cause of the fever, even if the eardrum is not red or bulging. This way, the doctor is able to end what otherwise might be a prolonged and perplexing search for a fever of unknown origin.

THE PARENT AS AN EAR EXAMINER ══

Many visits to a physician could be avoided if a parent could examine the child's eardrum at home and rule out the possibility of an ear infection. Although most parents would not want to depend upon their own ''diagnosis'' if a child is extremely ill, parents can learn to recognize the appearance of a healthy eardrum. It's gratifying to look in your child's ears with an otoscope and assure yourself that the child's irritability is not being caused by an ear infection, but probably by teething or fatigue.

Children who have their ears gently examined at home by parents may learn to sit still for a doctor during an office examination. A crying child is likely to have eardrums that look red and inflamed, which may lead to a misdiagnosis.

To learn how to diagnose ear infections, you must first know what you're looking for and be able to recognize changes in the eardrum which indicate infection. This book provides parents with a working knowledge of ear anatomy and descriptions and illustrations of the normal and abnormal eardrum.

Parents who learn how to use an otoscope may be able to save unnecessary trips to the physician in cases in which they're "not really sure" if the child is fussy because he has an ear infection or is fussy because he's teething or tired. Although the parent may never learn all the fine points of examining a child's ears, they can learn to tell the difference between a healthy and an inflamed eardrum. *(Photo by Cynthia J. Carney)*

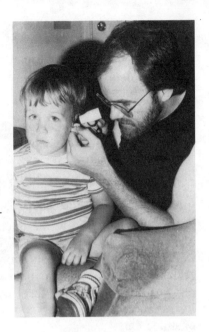

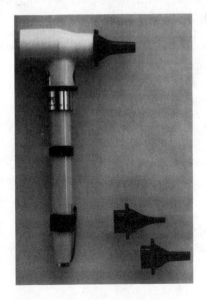

Parents can buy inexpensive otoscopes to examine their children's ears at home. Pictured here is the Earscope, a popular examining instrument for under $20.

Next, you must learn how to use an otoscope. Written descriptions and illustrations are no substitute for the actual experience of looking at the eardrum through the otoscope. It may take many attempts before you actually distinguish the eardrum from the ear canal, or learn to recognize when earwax is blocking the eardrum, but it's rewarding when you finally can detect abnormal findings such as a red, bulging eardrum or bubbles in middle ear fluid.

A doctor or nurse who is skilled at demonstrating the use of the otoscope is best qualified to teach and guide parents in examining each other and their children. With sufficient practice, a parent can gain enough confidence to determine when not to take the child to the doctor on the basis of his or her examination.

What kind of instruments should parents use at home? Several companies make inexpensive otoscopes designed especially for parents; two of these otoscopes are about $20.* The instrument comes with a very detailed explanation of how to examine ears.

If parents are interested in a better quality otoscope—that is, one that is not plastic and one that does not have a fixed focal length—they will have to pay more than $50. The Reister otoscope, an import from West Germany, is $55.* Higher quality otoscopes which are used in doctors' offices are much more expensive. However, some parents have pooled their resources to buy one good quality pneumatic otoscope and then share the instrument.

---

*"Earscope" can be ordered through Notoco, PO Box 300, Ferndale, CA 95536 or Cascade Birthing, PO Box 12203, Salem, OR 97309; the Reiser otoscope can be ordered through George Wootan, M.D., Box 101 K, RD7, Kingston, NY 12401.

QUESTIONS AND ANSWERS ▬▬▬▬

Q: My child has recurrent otitis media and his symptoms are unmistakable. If he has these symptoms, couldn't I just call my physician and ask him to prescribe antibiotics?

A: *Prescribing antibiotics over the phone without seeing a child is neither an accepted nor a common medical practice. The child could be experiencing another illness that is causing his discomfort, or the ear may have a condition that needs more serious and immediate treatment.*

Q: Can a physician determine if a child suffered an acute episode of otitis media, even if the symptoms have passed and the episode has subsided?

A: *Sometimes there are telltale signs that an ear infection has occurred, including an opaque but mobile eardrum, visible fluid or air bubbles in the fluid, or a retracted and pink eardrum.*

Q: Does an ear infection affect balance in a child?

A: *It may. Although there is no concrete evidence to establish the relationship, many parents have reported the combination. However, parents should know that dizziness and vertigo may indicate an inner ear infection. If your child has an ear infection and begins to fall when walking, or if he complains of dizziness, call your doctor immediately.*

Q: What is earwax?

A: *Earwax, medically known as cerumen, is glandular debris that accumulates in the ear canals, particularly if the canals are narrow or hairy. Cerumen provides a chemical barrier to infection and a mechanical barrier to foreign bodies.*

Q: Does earwax interfere with hearing? Does it ever build up to the point that it should be removed by a physician?

A: When wax totally occludes the ear canal, it may interfere with hearing and removal by a physician may be necessary.

Q: How can I tell the difference between earwax and drainage of the middle ear?

A: Earwax is oily and brownish. Drainage from the middle ear is sticky, yellowish or green, and may have a foul odor. Sometimes, melted earwax and draining middle ear pus look similar. A careful ear examination may be necessary to distinguish the two conditions.

Q: Should I remove wax from a child's ear?

A: If you can see the wax in the outer ear, it can be easily removed with a washcloth while bathing or washing the child. Parents who try to clean the ear with a cotton swab are only pushing the wax farther in toward the eardrum. Parents can also remove wax from children's ears by purchasing earwax removal drops and rubber bulb ear syringes, available over the counter in drug stores.

Q: If a child has pain or swelling behind his ear, how do you tell if it is an ear infection or a complication such as a mastoid infection?

A: An acute middle ear infection should not cause swelling behind the ear, but external ear infections can cause swelling around and behind the ear. Redness, tenderness, and a doughy swelling behind the ear could mean that mastoiditis is occurring.

Q: Does thick middle ear fluid cause more hearing loss or more problems than thin fluid? And how does the fluid get thick?

A: *Fluid thickness has no bearing on hearing.*[10] The fluid becomes thick as the body deposits sugars, white blood cells and other substances in the fluid.

Q: **Can my doctor examine the eustachian tube to find out if it is obstructed or not working properly?**

A: *In older and cooperative children, your doctor can use a mirror or a special telescope to examine the end of the eustachian tube and to see if the adenoid is blocking the eustachian tube. Also, a painless test can be done with a tympanometer (see Part Six for detailed discussion) to gain information about how well the eustachian tube is working. Sometimes your doctor may order an X-ray to see if the adenoid is large. The X-ray will show the size of the adenoid, but not if the adenoid is interfering with function of the eustachian tube.*

Q: **Does the otolaryngologist have special instruments which he can use to rid the eustachian tube of mucus?**

A: *Instruments to probe the opening of the eustachian tube and even to irrigate or force air into it are available. However, inserting these instruments into the end of the eustachian tube can be very uncomfortable for young children. Because of that—and because there are risks in doing the procedure— most doctors do not attempt to probe, irrigate or force air directly into the eustachian tubes of children.*

NOTES

1.   Schwartz, RH, Schwartz DM. Acute Otitis Media: Diagnosis and Drug Therapy. 1980: Drugs 19: 107–118.

1A.   Banco L. Earache As A Predictor of Acute Otitis Media in Children. AJDC. 1986 April: 140: 303.

2.   van Buchem FI, Dunk JHM, van't Hof MA. Therapy of acute

otitis media: Myringotomy, antibiotics or neither? Lancet 1981:883 –887.

3.   Diamant M, Diamant B. Abuse and timing of use of antibiotics in acute otitis media. Arch otolaryngol 1974; 100:226–232.

4.   Fry J. Antibiotics in acute tonsillitis and acute otitis media. Br Med J 1958; 883–886.

5.   Teele DW, Teele J. Detection of Middle Ear Effusion by Acoustic Reflectometry. The Journal of Pediatrics. 1984 June: 104(6): 832 –838.

6.   Lampe RM, Weir MR, Spier J, Rhodes MF. Acoustic Reflectometry in the Detection of Middle Ear Effusion. Pediatrics. 1985 July: 76(1):75–78.

7.   Schwartz DM, Schwartz RJ. Acoustic Reflectometry. Manuscript submitted for publication to Pediatrics.

8.   Mack RB. Do You Get Tensa when your house staff Cannot identify the flaccida? Presented at the Ambulatory Pediatric Association Meeting. 1984 Nov 3.

9.   Schwartz RH, Rodriguez WJ, McAveney W, Grundfast KM. Cerumen Removal, How Necessary Is It to Diagnose Acute Otitis Media? American Journal of Diseases of Children. 1983 Nov (137) 1064–1065.

10.   Marsh RR, Baranak CC, Potsic WP. Hearing loss and viscoelacticity of middle ear fluid. Int J Ped Otorhinolaryngology. 1985 July: 9(2): 115–120.

Problems That May Be Caused by Ear Infections

Today's generation of children is the first ever to receive aggressive treatment against ear infections, and many experts link that with the concurrent reduction in the number of serious, and sometimes fatal, illnesses caused by otitis media.

Many parents have a vague notion that untreated ear infections can lead to a dangerous disease. Often, these fears are heightened by a physician's stern warnings to administer the right amount of antibiotic, for the right number of days, or "the ear infection will get worse and spread." Other physicians, though still unclear, are more specific: "If you don't give your child antibiotics, he may develop meningitis or suffer permanent hearing loss."

These warnings can scare parents. Few serious illnesses, and far fewer deaths occur in the United States today as a result of otitis media. Otitis media is a self-limiting disease; that is, it will eventually subside if left untreated. The frequency of complications is about 5 percent today,[1] and although this low rate of serious disease is often attributed to aggressive treatment with antibiotics, even that link has not been firmly established.[2]

Physicians describe the adverse effects of certain diseases as "complications" or "sequelae." A complication is a disease occurring concurrently with another disease, such as otitis media. For example, mastoiditis is an infection of the mastoid bone that can occur along with an acute ear infection. A "sequelae" is an unwanted condition or illness that follows and is caused by some other disease. For example, on rare occasions, repeated ear infections can cause damage to the bones in the middle ear and impair hearing.

While complications rarely occur today except in neglected cases, sequelae are more common. Consequently, children are experiencing less serious conditions caused by persistent middle ear fluid, such as scarring of the eardrum. Although these sequelae are not life-threatening, they can cause temporary hearing loss, and if neglected, can damage structures in the middle ear.[1,3]

SEQUELAE

Thousands of children in the United States under age three have been treated for ear infections and suffer persistent middle ear fluid. Forty to 60 percent of children who have middle ear fluid probably will develop sequelae.[4] Even after the child no longer suffers from ear infections, some of the conditions resulting from otitis media persist for years. Rarely, sequelae can surface years following the child's last ear infection.

Researchers are uncertain if the increase in sequelae is actually a greater frequency of persistent middle ear effusion, or simply better detection of middle ear disease. Additionally, researchers are asking: Are the sequelae a result of the disease, or are they caused by today's aggressive treatment with antibiotics and insertion of ventilation tubes? What, if any, long-term effects will this treatment have on hearing and a child's entire ear structure?[3]

If your child's doctor mentions that he is concerned about a developing complication or sequelae in your child, ask him to fully explain to you the condition about which he is concerned, the reasons for the concern, and the recommended course to prevent further problems.

Physicians identify two kinds of sequelae: structural, which affects the middle ear bones or tissues; and developmental, which occurs when hearing loss causes speech and language delays or cognitive problems. Developmental problems are discussed thoroughly in Part Six; structural sequelae are described below:

Erosion of the ossicles. Like all bones in the body, the tiny middle ear ossicles (stapes, malleus and incus) require a blood supply for nourishment. When fluid remains in the middle ear for a prolonged time, the blood supply to the delicate ossicles can be restricted and erosion of portions of the ossicles can occur. Erosion can also be the result of pressure when an eardrum rests for a long time on a delicate portion of one of the ossicles.

Retracted eardrum (atelectasis). When the eustachian tube fails to function properly and negative pressure builds within the middle ear, the eardrum can lose some thickness and be sucked into the middle ear. If the eardrum can support the insertion of ventilation tubes, normal pressure can be restored within the middle ear.

Tympanosclerosis is characterized by chalky white plaques or deposits on the eardrum or in the middle ear and is most commonly found in older patients who suffered persistent middle ear fluid in their youth. Some studies have found the highest incidence among older patients who had ventilating tubes inserted as children.[4]

When the tympanosclerosis affects only the eardrum, little or no hearing loss is suffered and no specific treatment is warranted. At times, however, this condition can damage the ossicles and may cause hearing loss. Then, the plaques must be removed surgically.

Adhesive otitis media. Chronic inflammation can cause scars, called adhesions, to develop on the mucous membranes, ossicles or eardrum. If the adhesions are extensive and affect hearing, middle ear surgery may be necessary to repair the eardrum and reconstruct the ossicular chain.

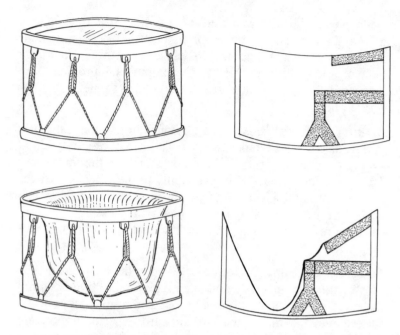

In these drawings, the eardrum is compared to the taut skin of a drum (top illustrations)—when it loses its tightness, the eardrum becomes slack and retracted and can rest on the middle ear ossicles.

Cholesteatoma occurs when an abnormal type of skin builds up behind the eardrum. This substance, which should be removed because it can harm the mastoid or the ossicles, is seen either as a white ball, or as white, shiny, greasy flakes of debris within an eardrum perforation or a sac in the eardrum. Sometimes, what appears to be a perforation in the eardrum can be a sac filled with the cholesteatoma.

How cholesteatoma develops is unknown. Some scientists believe that chronically inflamed and infected middle ear membranes undergo changes and form the debris. Another theory suggests that prolonged negative pressure in the middle ear weakens the eardrum, leading to the accumulation of the debris.[5]

Cholesteatoma can often be detected at an early enough

stage to allow preventive treatment. One patient visited an ENT specialist when a foul drainage from the ear occurred after an acute attack of otitis media. The specialist detected an abnormality on the eardrum and recommended the child be monitored closely over the next year. Treatment with ear drops cleared up the abnormality, but a year later, the doctor detected the early stages of cholesteatoma. Surgery was necessary to rebuild the eardrum and prevent the possible destruction.

COMPLICATIONS

Complications develop when an acute or chronic infection causes nearby bony structures to erode or break down. Bacteria then has a path into the inner ear, where it can attack the mastoid, or spread to the facial nerve. Perforation of the eardrum is the most common otitis media complication.

Serious complications from otitis media rarely occur in this country. For the most part, these occur in children who suffer frequently from acute otitis media and do not receive proper care.

Symptoms that indicate a serious problem may be developing are unmistakable and usually surface quickly and dramatically. Here are some typical complications:

Perforation of the eardrum. An eardrum can "burst" when a child has an ear infection. This can occur spontaneously during otitis media and is the body's way of draining the fluid that is bulging against the eardrum. A spontaneous perforation usually heals within 24 hours; if it doesn't, surgery may be required to repair the hole in the eardrum unless the perforation occurs in the young child who has frequent bouts of acute otitis media. Then, it can serve much the same function as a tympanostomy tube and surgery may be unnecessary.

Any perforation should be watched closely. If there is a persistent foul-smelling discharge from the ear, or if the physician observes flaky, whitish debris on the eardrum, a cholesteatoma may have developed.

Mastoiditis. The back wall of the middle ear has a small opening leading to the mastoid air cells (the mastoid is part of the temporal bone of the skull). In many cases of acute ear infections, the mastoid air cells become inflamed. Only in rare cases, however, does the inflammation become severe enough to be called mastoiditis. Symptoms associated with mastoiditis are redness, tenderness and bulging behind the ear, and high fever.

Labyrinthitis. This complication of otitis media occurs when infection spreads into the inner ear. Symptoms are vomiting, loss of hearing and loss of balance or vertigo.

Paralysis of the face. This condition develops when the facial nerve becomes inflamed and swollen.

Can Otitis Media Cause Meningitis?

Meningitis, an infection of the lining surrounding the brain, is a life-threatening illness. When a child develops an upper respiratory infection, the organism called Hemophilus influenzae can invade the membranes lining the nose and throat and gain access to the bloodstream. Once in the bloodstream, it can travel to the blood vessels in the lining surrounding the brain to cause meningitis.

A common concern among parents is that bacteria from an ear infection can spread into the brain and cause meningitis. In fact, this relationship has not been proven. A report in the *Journal of Pediatrics*[6] concluded that most children are not at risk to develop meningitis from acute otitis media. It also indicated that no pathway of infection could be found from the middle ear to the inner ear. The authors say that acute otitis media often accompanies an episode of meningitis, but that their "mutual presence might be coincidental."[6]

The authors also say that while a sharp decline in serious complications associated with acute otitis media has occurred, there has been a 400 percent increase in admissions to hospitals for meningitis over the past 25 years.[7,8] A new vaccine is being used to protect children against what physicians are calling the Hib (stands for the Hemophilus influenzae type b bacteria) disease. Hib is responsible in children for more than half of all cases of meningitis; more than 90 percent of epiglottis and a major portion of joint infections. This contagious disease[9] attacks one of every 200 children in the United States before age 5. However, the vaccine is not effective in preventing otitis media.

Even though there is no clear evidence showing that otitis media *causes* meningitis, a child with an upper respiratory infection and otitis media may develop meningitis as a result of bacteria that have circulated through the bloodstream. All parents should be familiar with early signs of meningitis, such as persistent high fever, headache, vomiting, stiff neck and lethargy or difficulty in arousing from sleep.

The relationship between acute otitis media and meningitis will continue to be explored by researchers in an effort to answer the following questions:

Does untreated acute otitis media put a child at risk for developing meningitis?

If a child is treated for 10 days with orally administered antibiotics for an ear infection, does this prevent the child from developing meningitis during and after completion of the antimicrobial therapy?

QUESTIONS AND ANSWERS ▅▅▅▅▅

Q: Sometimes my child does not show the classic signs of otitis media and acts fussy or clingy when she has an ear infection. Often, her eardrum had ruptured before I realized she had an acute infection. Is this frequent rupturing harmful to the eardrum?

A: Probably not. The eardrum usually heals quickly and can function normally after it heals. Remember, if your child is managing well without antibiotics or tubes, then periodic ear examination and assessment of hearing will assure that no harmful sequelae are developing.

Q: Can bacteria from a middle ear infection pass directly into the inner ear?

A: Some researchers postulate that middle ear fluid may pass through the round window membrane and damage sensory cells of the inner ear, leading to permanent hearing loss. Scientists are investigating the permeability of membranes in the round and oval windows to determine if, in fact, substances are able to pass from the middle ear and cause damage to the inner ear.[10]

NOTES

1.   Bluestone CD, Klein JO. "Otitis Media With Effusion, Atelectasis, and Eustachian Tube Dysfunction" in Pediatric Otolaryngology, Vol. 1. W.B. Saunders Co. 1983: p. 457.

2.   Gates GA. "Management" in Recent Advances in Otitis Media With Effusion (Lim DJ, editor). Annals of Otology, Rhinol and Laryngol. 1985 Jan–Feb: Suppl 116, 94 (1;3) 27–30.

3.   Paparella MM, Schachern PA. "Complications and Sequelae of Otitis Media: State of the Art" in Recent Advances in Otitis Media with Effusion (DJ Lim, Editor in Chief). B.C. Decker Inc., 1984: 316–319.

4.   Lim DJ. Aural Sequelae of Persistent Middle Ear Effusions. Pediatric Infectious Disease. Williams and Wilkins Co. 1982.

5.   Grundfast KM. "Diseases of the Ear" in Practice of Pediatrics (Kelley VC, editor). Harper & Row. Hagerstown, MD. 1980: Chapter 43, 1–41.

6.   Eavey RD, Gao YZ, Schuknecht HF, Gonzalez-Pineda M. Otologic Features of Bacterial Meningitis of Childhood. The Journal of Pediatrics. 1985 March: 106(3)402–406.

7.   Michaels RH: Increase in influenzal meningitis. N Engl J Med 285:666, 1971.

8.   Smith EWP Jr, Haynes RE. Changing incidence of Haemophilus influenzae meningitis. Pediatrics. 50:723, 1972.

9.   "A New Vaccine to Make the World a Safer Place For Your Child." Pamphlet distributed by Mead Johnson & Co. 1985. Evansville, Indiana 47721.

10.   Lim DJ, Chairman, "Anatomy, Cell Biology and Pathology" and Ruben RJ, Chairman, "Impact and Sequelae" Recent Advances in Otitis Media With Effusion (Lim DJ, editor). Annals Otology, Rhinology and L Laryngology. 1985 Jan–Feb:Suppl 116: 94(1:3):14–18 and 31–32.

PART TWO

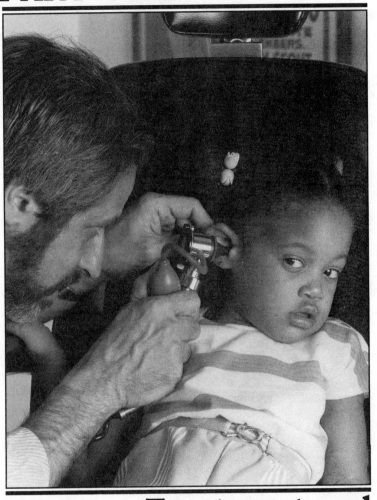

Treatment and Prevention

CHAPTER ONE

Goals
of Treatment

Philosophy of Treatment

Treatment of otitis media today is by no means uniform among physicians in the United States. Most treat the acute ear infection with antibiotics—but this is probably the only area with a relatively standard approach to treatment. If the child develops a chronic middle ear condition, what do most physicians do? And how effective are their courses of treatment?

The methods of treating persistent middle ear fluid are particularly controversial. Charles D. Bluestone, M.D., Professor of Otolaryngology, University of Pittsburgh School of Medicine and Director of Otolaryngology, Children's Hospital of Pittsburgh, is a leading expert on otitis media. He says:

Of the many methods of management that are available for otitis media with effusion, none has been shown to be effective in acceptable clinical trials. However, the clinician is forced to make a decision to treat actively or not to treat (watchful waiting); and if treatment is decided upon, which of the surgical or nonsurgical treatment options would be reasonable and most appropriate for the individual child.[1]

97

Questions abound: Should the physician take a "wait-and-see" approach? Should antibiotics be used to treat middle ear fluid? Is myringotomy effective in preventing middle ear fluid? How long should middle ear fluid be allowed to persist before tympanostomy tubes are inserted?

Even among otitis media experts, dissension is widespread, as characterized by this passage from a report summarizing the results of a conference of ENT specialists: "Passionate and stormy debate often made the deliberations of the panels painful. However, these debates stimulated thought and acquainted members with opposing opinions."[2]

Perhaps the most controversial of all reports was one conducted by researchers in the Netherlands.[3] In that study, four groups of children were treated by four different methods: neither antibiotics nor myringotomy; myringotomy only; antibiotics only; or both antibiotics and myringotomy. Researchers found no significant differences in the recovery rate among the four groups, and concluded myringotomy and antibiotics need not be used routinely in the treatment of acute otitis media. Three American physicians were skeptical about the results of the study because they found significant errors in the way the study had been designed and the data had been analyzed.[4]

Despite the controversy, the Dutch study challenged the medical community to reassess its routine and accepted treatments of otitis media. Significantly, it is only one of a number of studies—many of them conducted outside the United States—that question the standard practices of U.S. physicians. For instance, some experts suggest that antibiotics not be used routinely in the treatment of acute otitis media,[5,6] and when used, antimicrobial treatment can be limited to five or even two days rather than the customary 10 days.[7,8]

Goals of Treatment

The five middle ear conditions are listed below with a discussion of appropriate treatments.

The goals of treating *acute otitis media* are to relieve pain caused by infected fluid bulging against the eardrum and to relieve general symptoms such as fever; and to kill or inhibit growth of bacteria in the middle ear fluid. Methods to relieve pain include: administer non-aspirin liquid or tablet pain reliever; apply a warm towel or wash cloth to the infected ear to make child feel more comfortable; administer ear drops, such as Auralgan®; lance the eardrum (a procedure called myringotomy) to remove the fluid and resultant pressure; use antibiotics. To kill or remove bacteria: use antibiotics or perform myringotomy.

The presence of *middle ear fluid* is a normal consequence of an acute ear infection and, in most cases, will subside without treatment within six to eight weeks.[9] In many cases, the eardrum will not return to its normal appearance and fluid will continue to persist until two to three months have passed since the acute infection.[9]

Middle ear ventilation disorder, also known as a *retracted eardrum*, occurs when the eardrum is sucked into the middle ear cavity by a vacuum in the middle ear. Since no fluid or infection is present, the goal is to restore adequate aeration. Two treatment methods to restore air in the middle ear are (1) forcible aeration of the middle ear through the eustachian tube (methods described in next chapter); and (2) insertion of tympanostomy tubes to ventilate the middle ear through the eardrum.

Persistent middle ear fluid or frequently occurring acute otitis media: If your child's middle ear condition has been persisting for several months, you and your physician may meet to discuss what is causing the condition and what, if any, long-term treatment should be embarked upon. The physician has a responsibility not only to detect and diagnose the middle ear condition, but to uncover underlying causes. The treatment plan therefore must be directed at management of all conditions, including the causes as well as consequences.

Questions to discuss between you and your physician include:

- Is there an underlying cause such as allergy or abnormal palate? If so, can treatment be started to remedy the condition?

- Are other problems, such as hearing loss, developing as a result of the recurrent condition?

- Are there preventive measures that can be taken to help prevent the condition? This should include a discussion of the child's habits and stresses.

- Should an otolaryngologist (ear, nose and throat specialist) be consulted for possible surgical care?

Before the physician decides to refer a parent to an ENT specialist, he may consider: Taking a "wait-and-see" approach to see if the ear problems subside or prescribing a low dose of antibiotics over several months (prophylactic use of antibiotics) to clear up persistent middle ear fluid.

NOTES ════════════════════════════

1.   Bluestone CD. "Antimicrobial Therapy for Otitis Media With Effusion." Pediatric Annals. 1984 May: 13(5):405–410.
2.   Lim DJ, editor. Recent Advances in Otitis Media With Effusion. Introduction. Annals of Otology, Rhinology and Otolaryngology. 1985 Jan–Feb. Suppl. 116: 94 (1:3):6.
3.   van Buchem FI, Dunk JHM, van't Hof MA. Therapy of acute otitis media: Myringotomy, antibiotics or neither? Lancet 1981:883–887.
4.   Saah AJ. Letter. JAMA. 1982 Sept 3:248(9)1071.
5.   Paradise JL. "Otitis Media in Infants and Children." Pediatrics. 1980 May; 65 (5): 934.
6.   Diamant M, Diamant B. Abuse and timing of use of antibiotics in acute otitis media. Arch otolaryngol 1974; 100:226–232.
7.   Ingvarsson L; Lundgren K. "Penicillin treatment of acute otitis media in children. A study of the duration of treatment." Acta Otolaryngol (Stockh) 1982 Sep–Oct; 94 (3–4); 283–7.
8.   Meistrup-Larsen KI, et al. "Two versus seven days penicillin

treatment for acute otitis media. A placebo controlled trial in children." Acta Otolaryngol (Stockh) 1983 Jul–Aug; 96 (1–2): 99–104.

9.   Bluestone CD, Klein JO. "Otitis Media with Effusion, Atelectasis and Eustachian Tube Dysfunction" in Pediatric Otolaryngology Volume 1 (edited by CD Bluestone and SE Stool). 1983 WB Saunders Co.: 434.

Treatment at Home

Home Treatment of the Acute Ear Infection

When your child wakes up in the middle of the night screaming in pain from an ear infection, your only thought is to relieve the child's discomfort. The quickest and most effective ways to relieve pain at home are:

- Give the child a non-aspirin liquid or tablet pain reliever;
- Apply a warm towel or washcloth to the painful ear;
- Try to relax and calm the child so that he or she will sleep.

Auralgan®, a prescription ear drop, also can be used to help relieve the pain of an ear infection. Putting anything else in the ear to relieve pain such as olive oil may create a film over the eardrum and may prevent the physician from properly seeing the eardrum in order to make a diagnosis.

Knowing that the pain and fever of an acute ear infection will often subside within 24 hours, many parents will wait before taking the child to a doctor for examination. However, if the symptoms persist for more than 24 hours, the child should be examined by a physician. The physician may administer eardrops to numb the eardrum or may lance it to remove the pressure-causing fluid. Finally, the physician may prescribe antibiotics to relieve pain and treat the infection.

Treating the Acute Ear Infection at Home

- Give the child a non-aspirin pain reliever
- Apply warm towels to sore ear
- Relax, calm and comfort child
- Take child to emergency room only if child has high fever or other signs of severe illness, such as lethargy or inability to rouse

---

If It's an Emergency

If your child's pain seems quite severe and is not relieved by a pain reliever, then examination by a health professional is warranted since the pain may not be caused by a common ear infection. If you have difficulty contacting your child's doctor, or if the doctor seems reluctant to see your child after hours or on weekends, consider having your child's ears examined at an emergency room or at a 24-hour urgent care medical facility. If your child develops dizziness, vomiting, or a swelling behind the ear even after the pain is relieved, bring him to a doctor.

Forcing Air into the Middle Ear

If your child suffers persistent middle ear fluid or frequently occurring acute otitis media, chances are his eustachian tube is not opening and closing properly or that it is obstructed. When the eustachian tube does not ventilate the middle ear, a vacuum is created in the middle ear and fluid has no path from which to drain.

Can parents do anything to help ventilate their child's middle ear? The easiest way parents can help is by encouraging the

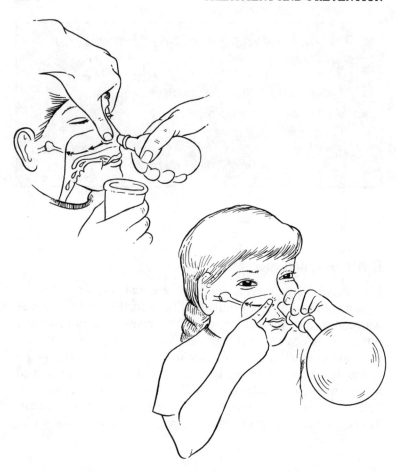

In the top illustration, the method of middle ear inflation shows a child taking a sip of water at the same time that air is being squeezed through an aspirator into one nostril, while the other nostril is pinched closed. As the child swallows the water, the eustachian tube opens. At the same time, the parent squeezes air through the aspirator and up through the eustachian tube. In the bottom illustration, the child pinches one of her nostrils shut while air is gently blown into her eustachian tube as the air flows out of the inflated balloon. In this instance, the child can say "cookie, cookie, cookie" or "kay, kay, kay" to open the eustachian tube.

child to swallow more frequently and open his mouth wide by chewing gum or sucking on a pacifier or teething toy. By swallowing more frequently, the eustachian tube will open more frequently.

However, methods to force air into the middle ear are more sophisticated and complicated than swallowing. These methods date back to the early 1700s when Antonio Valsalva, who held the Chair of Anatomy in Bologna, located and named the eustachian tube.[1] Through the centuries, as the function of the eustachian tube was studied, more methods to force air into the middle ear were developed. Adam Politzer in the early part of this century developed a techique by which an India-rubber air bag pressed air into the middle ear through a catheter inserted into the opening of the eustachian tube in the throat. A modified version of Politzer's technique is still used today.

The various techniques of forcing air into the middle ear through the eustachian tube are not used as frequently today because of the widespread use of ventilation tubes. But, there are practical reasons for eschewing the aeration techniques. First, and most important, the methods cannot be used while the child has a cold, because they can force bacteria or viruses into the middle ear. Second, most children do not tolerate the techniques until at least age 4; not only do the techniques require cooperation and physical coordination of the child, they produce a startling popping sensation in the ears if the method is successful. Third, in order for the aeration techniques to effectively clear middle ear fluid, they should be performed on the child at least three times a day for as long as several weeks.[2]

Despite the obstacles associated with forced-air techniques, they are included as a possible way to help ventilate the middle ear. David Fairbanks, M.D., a Washington, D.C., ENT specialist reports that one-half to two-thirds of children who have had persistent middle ear fluid have been able to clear the condition after practicing the techniques on a regular basis. Fairbanks says the techniques are an alternative to inserting tympanostomy tubes.[2]

Three methods of aerating the middle ear are:

Toynbee maneuver (the least forceful method). Swallow while the nostrils are pinched shut or swallow simultaneously while blowing against closed nostrils.

Politzerization (modified version). An infant nasal aspirator is inserted into one nostril, the other nostril is pinched shut, and the child is instructed to take a sip of water while the parent squeezes air through the nose. Though not as effective, the child can say "cookie, cookie" or "kaykaykay" while the air is blown into the nose, instead of taking a sip of water.

Middle ear inflator. The Mathes Inflator® is a balloon-like inflation device that many parents and children have found to be simpler than the traditional Politzerization technique. The parent inflates the balloon, applies the nozzle to one nostril, pinches close the other nostril and allows the balloon to deflate as the child swallows a sip of water or says "cookie, cookie" or "kaykaykay." (The Mathes Middle Ear Inflator® can be ordered for $5 plus postage through Almat Inc., PO Box 3220, Johnson City, TN 37601.)

There is probably no effective "trick" to elicit cooperation from your child in using these methods. Some parents make a game of it and suggest the balloon is like a spaceship taking off, or talk about it in positive terms, like, "Let's pop our ears now!"

Decongestants/Antihistamines

An antihistamine dries the nasal passages by blocking the effect of histamine, a substance that causes congestion and which is released during an allergic reaction. A decongestant, such as Novafed® or Sudafed®, also has a drying effect on the nasal passages. Neither medication has been shown to affect the eustachian tube or middle ear function or alter the course of otitis media.[3] Nonetheless, physicians continue to prescribe either, or a combination of both for children who have a runny nose accompanying an ear infection. The physicians believe by relieving nose congestion, there is less chance that infected mucus can travel through the eustachian tube to the middle ear. Although antihistamines and decongestants can relieve stuffiness and make the child more comfortable, parents should realize that the medication is treating the congestion accompanying a cold and not the ear infection.

Some unwanted side effects may accompany these medications. Drowsiness is a common side effect of antihistamines, but the reverse is also possible: they can stimulate the central nervous system and cause restlessness.[4] The decongestant is a stimulator which can override this drowsy effect. Besides altering the blood pressure, these medications may harm the cilia of the nasal passages and the eustachian tube.[4]

Nose drops also can be prescribed to relieve nasal congestion. However, using the nose drops for more than five days can harm the tissues in the nose and sinuses.

For a child who has allergies, decongestants or antihistamines may relieve constant stuffiness. However, some physicians think it unwise to recommend either medication for infants and children because of the potentially harmful effects.

Other Medications

One substance that has been tested infrequently in the treatment of otitis media is called an oral mucolytic agent and which has been found to reduce the thickness of mucus in chronic chest diseases. Researchers thought the agent might act as a thinning agent in persistent middle ear fluid. An Australian study showed the use of such an agent, called bromhexine, helped clear middle ear fluid 3.6 times more often than a group treated with placebos.[5] However, this study is only the first in many that must prove the mucolyctic's efficacy in treating otitis media.

Corticosteroid, in a spray or oral form, is another substance that has been used in the treatment of otitis media. Some researchers speculate that this medication, derived from the hormone prednisone, helps shrink swollen tissue in the eustachian tube and decreases the thickness of the fluid in the middle ear. However, studies on the effects of corticosteroid in the treatment of otitis media do not yet warrant its use in treating or preventing otitis media.[6]

NOTES

1.   Pahor AL. An Early History of Secretory Otitis Media. The Journal of Laryngology and Otology. 1978 July: 543–560.
2.   Fairbanks DN, Webb BM. Eustachian Tube Inflation in the Treatment of Middle Ear Fluid. Clinical Proceedings, Children's Hospital National Medical Center.
3.   Cantekin EI, et al. Lack of Efficacy of a Decongestant-Antihistamine Combination for Otitis Media with Effusion ("Secretory" Otitis Media) in Children. New England Journal of Medicine. 1983 Feb. 10: 308(6):297–301.
4.   Roundtable discussion. "Otitis Media: Selecting the Therapy." Patient Care. 1983 Sept. 15:17(15):108–146.
5.   Roydhouse N. "Bromhexine in the Treatment of Otitis Media with Effusion" in Recent Advances in Otitis Media with Effusion (DJ Lim, senior editor). 1984: B.C. Decker: 266–268.
6.   Bluestone CD, Klein JO. "Otitis Media with Effusion, Atelectasis and Eustachian Tube Dysfunction" in Pediatric Otolaryngology Volume 1 (edited by CD Bluestone and SE Stool). 1983 WB Saunders Co.: 470.

CHAPTER THREE

Treating the Allergic Child

Is There a Link Between Allergy and Otitis Media?

Scientists are unsure if allergies cause otitis media, but many studies have shown that children who suffer frequent nasal congestion because of allergies may be more prone to ear infections than allergy-free children.[1,2,3] Therefore, controlling the allergy—which diminishes nasal and eustachian tube congestion—may help decrease frequently occurring otitis media and/or persistent middle ear fluid. This section is only an introduction to allergy identification and management. For more information, consult the following books:

- *Parents Book of Childhood Allergies* by Richard F. Graber, Ballantine Books, 1983.

- *The Complete Book of Children's Allergies: A Guide for Parents* by Robert Feldman and David Carroll, Times Books, 1982.

- *Tracking Down Hidden Food Allergy* by William G. Crook, Prof Bks Future Health, 1980.

What Is Allergy?

The allergic person is overly sensitive to certain substances in the air or food. The body reacts to these substances as it would to any invasion of disease—by rallying its defenses to fight infection; specifically, the body releases antibodies (known as the substance IgE) which become "fixed" to the mucus membranes of the nose and which release histamines. The histamines cause dilation of the blood vessels, stimulate the production of mucus and produce other changes in the body to ward off the offending substance. As a result, the allergic person has symptoms such as stuffiness, headache, sneezing, tiredness and circles under the eyes.

Diagnosing Allergy and Identifying Allergic Substances

Because many children have runny noses all winter long, parents often surmise that the constant congestion is being caused by an allergy. However, a continually runny nose is common for many children under age four and does not necessarily indicate an allergy. Most children have an average of five colds during a winter season. If other symptoms accompany the congestion, such as sneezing, red and watery eyes, dark circles under the eyes, and irritability, then your child may have an allergy. Consult an allergist if your child suffers the symptoms just described, or if continual congestion and recurrent middle ear problems have not cleared up by the age of four.

An allergist will test your child and identify the substances causing allergic reactions. Among other tests, the allergist will evaluate antibody function with blood tests and will inject allergic substances into the skin to try to elicit allergic reactions.

Removing Allergic Substances From the Home

Treating the allergic child may be as simple as eliminating offending substances from the home. For instance, if the child is allergic to pets, they should be removed from the house. The most important room in controlling allergic substances is the child's bedroom: stuffed toys should be removed; floors should be bare of carpets; pillows, sheets and bedspreads containing fluffy material should be avoided; and walls, windows and furniture should be cleaned frequently.

During the winter months when the furnace is operating, the air in the house may become very dry. A central humidifier can help boost the humidity to a preferred 30 to 40 percent.[2] Frequent changing of the furnace filter may aid in removing large particles of house dust. Also, if the child is allergic to pollens, air conditioning may be used during the summer. A child may be discouraged from spending time in any area (such as a basement) that may be moldy or chilly; but dampness can be controlled somewhat by a dehumidifier.

Removing Allergic Foods From the Diet

Your child may exhibit allergic reactions, such as nasal stuffiness, dark circles under the eyes, sneezing or skin rashes after eating certain foods. You can test for such allergies with an "elimination" diet. For example, if you suspect that milk is causing the reaction, remove it and other milk products from the child's diet for a week; then, on the eighth day, let the child drink large amounts of milk. If a reaction occurs, your child likely is allergic to milk and dairy products.

An elimination diet can be done in the reverse manner by eliminating everything except one or two basic foods, and then reintroducing a new food every week. This severe form of the elimination diet is used with children who are suspected of being allergic to many kinds of food. Milk and dairy products such as cheese are the most common sources of food allergies in children. One study showed that the elimination of foods traditionally shown to cause allergy helped reduce otitis media in allergic children.[4]

Using Medication to Relieve Allergic Symptoms

Antihistamines and decongestants may help relieve the stuffiness of nasal congestion due to allergy, but they have not been proven to alter the course of otitis media (see preceding chapter for discussion of antihistamines and decongestants).

Nose drops and sprays and steroid aerosols help control nasal congestion, but should be used for only a limited amount of time, especially in children, because they may harm nasal tissues.

Antibiotics should be used only when a bacterial infection is present; they are not useful in relieving congestion or allergic symptoms, such as a swollen eustachian tube.

Immunotherapy (allergy shots) is used to treat patients who are allergic to airborne substances, such as pollen, molds and house dust. This therapy, called hyposensitization or desensitization, is administered through a series of injections that stimulate the production of a "blocking antibody" (IgG), which protects the individual when he's exposed to the airborne substance.

NOTES ══════════════════════════════

1.   Curtis AW, Clemis JD. "Middle Ear Effusions: Part 1—Pathophysiology." The Journal of Continuing Education in O.R.L. and Allergy. 1979 May: 13–25.
2.   Miller DL, Friday GA. Allergic Diseases of the Nose and Middle Ear in Children. Ear, Nose and Throat Journal. 1978 March; 57; 27–115.
3.   Bluestone CD, Klein JO. "Otitis Media with Effusion, Atelectasis and Eustachian Tube Dysfunction" in Pediatric Otolaryngology Volume 1 (edited by CD Bluestone and SE Stool). 1983 WB Saunders Co.: 472.
4.   Ruokonen J, Paganus A, Lehti H. Elimination diets in the treatment of secretory otitis media. Int J Pediatr Otorhinol. 1982 May:4(1):39–46.

CHAPTER FOUR

Prevention

One mother was dismayed when an ENT specialist told her the only way to prevent her child from getting another ear infection was to keep him at home and away from other children. Another ENT specialist suggested that she and her husband wear masks around their child when one or the other had a cold.

Certainly, these measures may seem severe: a child's life cannot stand still because he has recurrent ear infections; and when he is healthy, it is important for him to socialize with his peers and to accompany his parent or caretaker in the daily routine. And, sick or not, the child deserves loving care uninhibited by a parent afraid of infecting, or getting infected by, a child.

A child's middle ear is extremely susceptible to infection because of its proximity to the upper respiratory tract. Many children go through an entire winter season with a runny nose, and it is not uncommon for a runny nose to lead to an ear infection. Therefore, it's important to keep your child's illnesses in perspective: a child who has four or five ear infections in one winter season should not be considered a sickly or ill child.

Short of isolation, what can you do to prevent ear infections in the child who is prone to them? Unfortunately, there are no foolproof measures to prevent colds and ear infections. However, some basic guidelines are helpful:

Practices at Home

Infants and toddlers should not be put to bed with bottles, since the liquid could be sucked up into the eustachian tube and lead to an ear infection (see explanation of bottle propping on page 49).

Nutrition

Breastfeeding may play an important role in protecting the infant from illness and in delaying the onset of a child's first ear infection. One study showed a greater frequency of viral and upper respiratory infections in bottle fed infants as compared to those breastfed in the first six months of life. These researchers concluded that breastfeeding for at least three months may enhance an infant's immune competence, thereby improving his ability to fight ear infections.[1] In a second study, no breastfed baby developed otitis media before the age of six months.[2] Yet another study showed breastfeeding had a long-term protective effect for up to three years; the longer the child was breastfed, the fewer episodes of otitis media. However, early weaning to a cow's milk formula was correlated with increases in the number of episodes of otitis media.[3]

Vaccines

Immunization against disease has played a vital part in the battle against such enemies as tetanus, smallpox and polio. The body creates an antibody to a disease when a foreign substance (called an antigen) invades the body. A vaccination artificially creates this immune response by injecting the individual with a serum of antigenic material.

Scientists remain hopeful that a vaccine can be created to prevent children from developing otitis media. One vaccine, called the pneumococcal polysaccharide vaccine, has been used successfully in the prevention of pneumonia in adults. Since many cases of acute otitis media are caused by pneumococci, the National Institute of Allergy and Infectious Disease in 1974 began trials of the vaccine to prevent otitis media in childhood.[4]

To date, the vaccine has not been shown to be of significant value in management of children with middle ear infections.[5] The major drawback to the vaccine is that it is ineffective in children under two years of age, because their ability to produce antibody is not mature enough to mount a strong response. Several studies have shown that the vaccine can offer up to 50 percent protection against the disease in older children, but only 10 percent protection against overall incidence of otitis media; also, it's not known how long the vaccine is effective.[6]

A new vaccine, called Hib for the Hemophilus influenzae type b bacteria, has not been shown to be effective in preventing otitis media. The Hib vaccine is used against illnesses in children such as meningitis, epiglottis and joint infections (see page 92).

Treating the Allergy May Prevent the Ear Infection

If your child wheezes, sneezes frequently, has a continually runny nose and watery or red eyes, or has dark circles under his eyes, you may want to consult an allergist to determine if his nasal congestion is caused by an allergy. You may be able to help reduce incidences of otitis media by eliminating the allergic substance from the child's environment or diet. (See preceding chapter for complete discussion of treating the allergic child.)

Ventilating the Middle Ear

Although techniques for forcibly aerating the middle ear are included as a treatment on pages 104–106, parents also may use these measures to improve aeration of a child's ear and perhaps diminish its tendency to infection. The child who constantly has a vacuum (negative pressure) in the middle ear is likely to have frequent ear discomfort and repeated ear infections. Although there are no scientific studies to prove or disprove the notion, it is logical to assume improved aeration of the middle ear can reduce a child's tendency to develop ear infections.

Prophylactic Antibiotics

A daily, small dose of antibiotics may help diminish the frequency of acute otitis media and may clear up middle ear fluid. The use of antibiotic in this preventative, or prophylactic, way is discussed in Part Four.

Surgical Measures to Prevent Otitis Media

Myringotomy with insertion of tympanostomy tubes as a measure to reduce the number of episodes of acute otitis media and to help clear middle ear fluid is discussed in Part Five. Another surgical measure that can be considered is adenoidectomy, which is discussed in Part Three.

The Hardest Battle to Fight:
The Common Cold

Many children frequently develop otitis media after a bout with a cold. Preventing and curing the common cold in young children is impossible. There is no medication or method proven to prevent the ear infections associated with colds; however, the following guidelines may be helpful when your child has a cold:

Keep the child at home for several days of quiet play and make sure he gets plenty of rest and fluids.

Keep his nose as clear as possible. For children who are too young to blow their own noses, use an aspirator to clear the mucus.

Some physicians recommend a *vaporizer* to help liquify mucus. However, it should be used in moderation because excessive humidity could create a damp, humid environment which can foster the growth of mold on the walls.

To help move mucus out of the chest, turn on all the hot water faucets in a closed bathroom and *create a sauna effect.* After the child has inhaled this steam for 10–15 minutes, lay him on his stomach and pat gently on his back with cupped hands to help break up the mucus in his lungs.

Some Final Words of Encouragement

Remember, a child's defenses against disease are still maturing during the first five years of life. These defenses, called the immune system, are affected by many environmental factors such as nutrition, fatigue and emotional stress, as well as by biological factors such as heredity. Despite the fact that ear infections in childhood are frequent and annoying, they are rarely dangerous or harmful. Although there may be little that you can do to prevent the ear infections, take some solace by remembering your child will outgrow the problem. If you make every attempt to comfort your child when ear pain develops, to seek medical attention when needed, and to monitor hearing ability and speech development, then you are doing everything possible to provide the best care for your child.

NOTES

1. Persico M, Podoshin L, et al. Recurrent Middle Ear Infections in Infants: The Protective Role of Maternal Breastfeeding. Ear, Nose and Throat Journal. 1983 June:20–31.
2. Breastfeeding Prevents Otitis Media. Nutrition Review. 1983 Aug:41(8)241–2.
3. Prolonged Breastfeeding as Prophylaxis for Recurrent Otitis Media. Acta Pediatric Scan. 1982 July:71(4):567–71.
4. Hill JC. "Immunization Against Pneumococcal Otitis Media: State of the Art" in Recent Advances in Otitis Media With Effusion (DJ Lim, senior editor). 1984: B.C. Decker: 249–250.

5. Hill JC. "Special Remarks" in Recent Advances in Otitis Media With Effusion. Annals of Otology, Rhinology and Laryngology. 1985 Jan–Feb: Suppl. 116: 94(1:3) 7.

6. Hill JC. "Immunization Against Pneumococcal Otitis Media: State of the Art" in Recent Advances in Otitis Media With Effusion (DJ Lim, Editor in Chief). B.C. Decker Inc., 1984: 249–251.

PART THREE

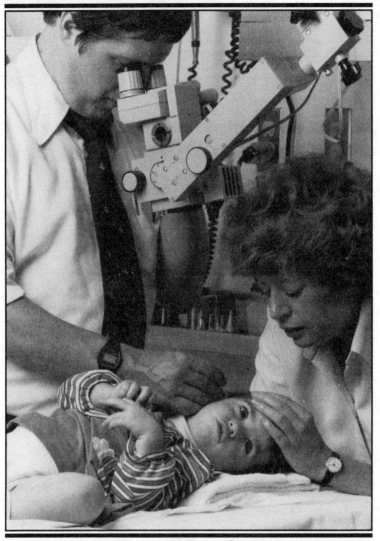

Myringotomy
and Other Surgery

Myringotomy and Other Surgery

MYRINGOTOMY

A myringotomy is performed by making a small incision in the eardrum with a surgical knife. The procedure is similar to the lancing of a boil to release infected fluid under pressure. The fluid is either allowed to drain out by itself, or is aspirated with a suction instrument. The myringotomy incision usually heals within 24 to 48 hours without any adverse affects.

The incision may be only the size of a pinprick or a few millimeters in length. If the eardrum is bulging and red with thickened pus pressing against it, the incision must be larger to allow the pus to escape; if the fluid is clear and thin, the incision can be quite small.

When a physician aspirates middle ear fluid through an opening made with a needle, it's called tympanocentesis. The fluid then can be sent to a laboratory for analysis to determine the type of bacteria that caused the infection and to test the effectiveness of certain antibiotics against that bacteria. This is called "culture and sensitivity" testing.

Purposes of Myringotomy

Myringotomy can provide immediate relief from the pressure and pain of an ear infection. Some primary care physicians

121

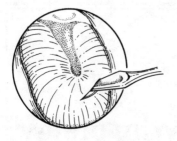

Myringotomy is performed with a tiny surgical knife. The physician makes a small incision to allow fluid that is trapped behind the eardrum to escape through the ear canal.

and ENT specialists use it routinely to treat infants with intense ear pain and high fever.

Myringotomy can also be used to drain and obtain a sample of middle ear fluid from a child who has not responded to antimicrobial treatment or who is on antibiotics for the treatment of another condition.

Finally, some physicians use myringotomy in cases of persistent middle ear fluid that have not responded to a course of antimicrobial treatment.

Where and How Is Myringotomy Performed?

Myringotomy usually is performed in a physician's office and takes no more than a few minutes after the child has been restrained and the physician has prepared the necessary instruments. The actual process of making the incision is very brief: The surgeon first will clean wax from the ear canal, sterilize the area with alchohol or an iodine solution, and make a tiny incision in the eardrum.

For a very young child, the procedure is uncomfortable because he must be immobilized (usually by a papoose), he feels some pressure, and the incision itself is momentarily painful. If an aspirator is used to drain the fluid, the child may be frightened by its loud noise.

Though most myringotomies are performed without local anesthesia, a method is available for desensitizing the eardrum without needles or injections. This procedure, called iontophoresis, consists of dropping an anesthetic liquid into the ear

Purposes of Myringotomy

- To provide immediate relief from pain of ear infection
- Drain middle ear fluid from child whose acute infection has not responded to antibiotic
- Drain fluid from child whose chronic ear problems have not responded to prophylactic antimicrobial treatment

canal and drawing the liquid into the eardrum battery-operated device that emits a low level electrical current. The child must lie still for 10 minutes for this method to be successful.

A properly-performed myringotomy should present few risks, but there is always the remote possibility that the wrong area of the eardrum could be incised, or that the ossicles could be damaged with a slip of the knife.

Taking a New Look at an Old Practice

Myringotomy was the only procedure used before the advent of antibiotics to relieve pressure and pain from otitis media. Because of its therapeutic importance, physicians of a generation or more ago routinely learned how to perform a my-

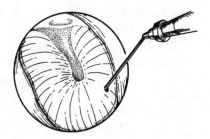

This process is called tympanocentesis. A hollow needle is inserted into the eardrum to aspirate fluid from the middle ear.

ringotomy; some of these physicians still continue to use myringotomy in the routine care of otitis media.

Today, however, training programs for pediatricians do not routinely teach this skill and pediatric residents often do not learn it. Myringotomy is used less often now than previously because it has been displaced by antibiotic therapy, which is less complicated to administer; many cases of acute otitis media resolve without treatment; and many physicians who provide primary care to children are not comfortable performing the procedure.

However, because of the recent increase in chronic middle ear problems among children, myringotomy's efficacy is being reevaluated by many experts, and studies are now determining if myringotomy has a place in management of chronic middle ear conditions. Charles D. Bluestone, M.D., and Jerome Klein, M.D., state in the textbook *Pediatric Otolaryngology*:

> *The potential benefit from more liberal use of the procedure in cases of acute otitis media might be relief of ear pain and a decrease in persistence and recurrence rates. When chronic otitis media with effusion is present, myringotomy may be equally as effective in eliminating the middle ear fluid as when procedure is followed by insertion of a tympanostomy tube.*[1]

Other experts in childhood otitis media believe myringotomy is underused, and that the general practitioner and pediatrician should be able to perform this office procedure quickly, routinely and efficiently. Two other experts discuss the infrequent use of myringotomy today:

George Gates, M.D., head of the division of otolaryngology at the Department of Surgery, University of Texas Health Science Center in San Antonio believes myringotomy is underused. "The absence of training in this technique in pediatric residents is not in the best interests of patients with severe acute otitis media."[2]

Jack L. Paradise, M.D., Pittsburgh Children's Hospital,

says the more liberal use of myringotomy in the treatment of acute otitis media is promising and advocates study of myringotomy as a measure to prevent chronic ear infections.[3]

Heat Myringotomy

Heat, or thermal, myringotomy using a commercially available, battery-powered device can make an incision in the eardrum that remains open for one to three weeks. The instrument used to perform this procedure, called Thermo-Vent®, burns a hole in the eardrum with a hot wire tip after the eardrum has been anesthesized. A trigger on the device activates a timed power pulse that shuts off automatically in three seconds. An advantage to this procedure is that it can be done in the doctor's office without using general anesthesia, and could possibly be used as an alternative to insertion of tympanostomy tubes.[4]

ADENOIDECTOMY AND/OR TONSILLECTOMY

Adenoids and tonsils are growths of lymphoid tissue in the part of the throat behind the nose and mouth that help trap particles and destroy bacteria and viruses entering the nose and mouth. The adenoids are located in the upper part of the throat, behind the nose; the tonsils are a pair of oval masses situated each side of the throat at the back of the mouth. When infected, the adenoids can swell up and obstruct parts of the nasopharyngeal passage. In the 1940s and 1950s, tonsillectomies were performed on thousands of children in an effort to prevent strep throats and upper respiratory infections. The adenoids were often removed during the same operation. Over the last 15 years, the number of tonsillectomies has declined dramatically.

No controlled scientific study has proven that the removal of tonsils or adenoids prevents otitis media.[5] In recent years, although, more attention has been paid to the therapeutic benefit of adenoidectomy in preventing otitis media, no conclusive data are yet available. Current studies are being conducted at the Children's Hospital of Pittsburgh and the University of Texas Health Science Center at San Antonio.[6]

Adenoidectomy, either separately or with tonsillectomy, is the most common major surgical procedure among children, and is often performed by otolaryngologists who believe that the operation helps prevent otitis media.[5] Still, the number of adenoidectomies being done each year in the United States is declining. In 1965, 981,000 children under the age of 15 underwent surgery for adenoidectomy and tonsillectomy; by 1986, that number had been reduced by 85.32 percent to 144,000. Only 14,000 children in 1986 underwent adenoictomy alone; and 33,000 underwent tonsillectomy alone.[6] (See Chart 2 on page 9.)

NOTES ══════════════════════════

1. Bluestone CD, Klein JO. "Otitis Media with Effusion, Atelectasis and Eustachian Tube Dysfunction" in *Pediatric Otolaryngology* Volume 1 (edited by CD Bluestone and SE Stool). 1983 WB Saunders Co.: 476.

2. Gates GA. The Role of Myringotomy in Acute Otitis Media. Pediatric Annals. 1984 May;13(5): 391–397.

3. Paradise JL. On Tympanostomy Tubes: Rationale, Results, Reservations and Recommendations. Pediatrics. 1977 July: 60 (1): 86–90.

4. Lau P, Goode RL, et al. Heat Myringotomy. Laryngoscope. 1985 Jan: 95: 38–41.

5. Gates, GA. Effect of adenoidectomy upon children with chronic otitis media with effusion. Laryngoscope. 1988 Jan; 98 (1): 58-63. Also, Gates GA. Effectiveness of adenoidectomy and tympanostomy tubes in the treatment of chronic otitis media with effusion. New England J of Medicine. 1987 Dec 3;317(23): 1444-51.

6. Information based on list of CRISP records of currently active USPHS grants and contracts and NIH intramural projects active in 1984 from the Division of Research Grants, Department of Health and Human Services, Public Health Service.

7. Hospital Discharge Survey, National Center for Health Statistics, unpublished data.

PART FOUR

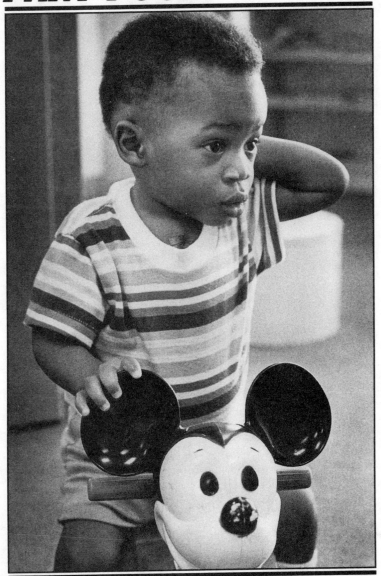

Antibiotics

Antibiotics

What Are Antibiotics and How Do They Work?

Antibiotics are naturally-occurring or synthetically-made chemical substances that destroy bacteria or inhibit their growth. An oral dose of antibiotics is absorbed into the bloodstream and circulated throughout the body. The blood vessels carry some of the antibiotic to the middle ear space, where it mixes with the fluid containing bacteria. If the antibiotic works properly, the bacteria begin to die and the infection and related symptoms of pain and fever will subside within a few hours.

"Resistant" Bacteria

Each type of antibiotic is effective on specific types of bacteria and no single antibiotic is effective for all ear infections all of the time. When a bacteria can be killed by an antibiotic, it is said to be "susceptible" to that antibiotic; conversely, if a bacteria remains alive in the presence of an antibiotic, the bacteria is "resistant" to it. Therefore, if a child's symptoms of severe ear pain and high fever are not relieved within 24 hours after the first dose of the antibiotic, the bacteria may be resistant to the antibiotic.

When an antibiotic is commonly used over many years in

a region of a country, new strains of bacteria may develop to cause otitis media which will be resistant to those common antibiotics. This rise in bacterial resistance to antibiotics is attributed to the frequent use of antibiotics in the treatment of otitis media.[1]

What to Expect From Antimicrobial Treatment

You will know an antibiotic is doing its job if your child's acute symptoms such as ear pain, fever and irritability are gone within 24 hours after the first dose. The only realistic expectations of antimicrobial therapy are that bacteria are killed, and therefore, symptoms are relieved.

Many parents believe that an antibiotic "cures" an ear infection. Although the antibiotic does speed up the body's healing processes by killing bacteria, the body's immune system ultimately must return the middle ear to normal, a process which may take two to three months before the eardrum returns to its normal appearance and all fluid disappears.[2] Antibiotics do not automatically make the middle ear fluid disappear; they may not kill all the bacteria; and they do not immediately restore the eardrum to its normal appearance.

Antibiotic Treatment

What to Expect from Antibiotic

- Kills most bacteria, thereby relieving pain

What Not to Expect From Antibiotic

- Doesn't clear up middle ear fluid immediately
- May not kill all bacteria
- Does not restore eardrum to normal appearance

How Does Doctor Choose Antibiotics?

- Age of child
- Allergies to antibiotics
- Physician's preference

How Does My Doctor Choose the "Right" Antibiotic?

Physicians cannot know exactly what organism is causing otitis media unless they aspirate the middle ear fluid and "culture" it. Therefore, a physician considers several factors before prescribing an antibiotic to treat otitis media, including:

Age of the child. Bacteria that cause middle ear infections in infants less than six weeks of age may not be the common variety of organisms. Therefore, some physicians routinely prick the eardrum with a hollow needle and aspirate middle ear fluid (called tympanocentesis) to determine precisely which bacteria are causing the ear infection. Tympanocentesis also is used routinely in the treatment of newborns because of the difficulty of diagnosis (their ear canals are small and undeveloped). The sample of middle ear fluid is sent to a laboratory for bacteriologic testing, called "culture and sensitivity" testing.

Allergies. If a child has previously had an allergic reaction to an antibiotic, an alternative antibiotic will be prescribed.

Physician's preference. A physician may prefer a certain antibiotic, especially if some antibiotics have been shown to be ineffective in treating otitis media in that region of the country. Also, once a physician learns all the dosage forms and side effects of a certain medication, he may become comfortable with the medication and prescribe it often.

Antibiotics Used in the Treatment of Otitis Media

In the last 10 years, pharmaceutical manufacturers have marketed new kinds of antibiotics in response to the demand for medication to treat otitis media. The liquid forms of these antibiotics have been created with children in mind; many are fruit flavored. At least one antibiotic—Pediazole®—was manufactured specifically to treat otitis media and another antibiotic—Augmentin®—was manufactured to fight strains of bacteria that are resistant to amoxicillin.[3]

The most common "families" of antibiotics used in the treatment of otitis media are the penicillins, the cephalosporins, the sulfonamides (usually combined with trimethoprim, such as Bactrim® and Septra®) and erythromycin (combined with sulfisoxazole to make Pediazole®). These antibiotics have been determined to be effective in killing the two most common forms of bacteria that cause otitis media: Hemophilus influenzae and Streptococcus pneumoniae.

Antibiotics used in the treatment of otitis media are described below:

Amoxicillin. The most commonly prescribed antibiotic used to treat ear infections, amoxicillin (a generic name) is a semisynthetic penicillin. Amoxicillin consistently has been shown to be the most effective antibiotic in combatting bacteria usually found in ear infections.[4] It is estimated that in 1984, amoxicillin was prescribed in 39 percent of office visits to treat otitis media.[5]

Physicians favor amoxicillin because it is given only three times a day, is absorbed well in the gastrointestinal tract, and is less likely to cause diarrhea than some other antibiotics.[4] Some physicians use ampicillin, which is similar to amoxicillin, to treat otitis media.

Pediazole®. A combination of erythromycin and sulfisoxazole, Pediazole® can be used if a child is allergic to penicillin.

Bactrim® **and** *Septra*®. A combination of trimethoprim and sulfamethoxazole, these drugs are alternatives for children who are allergic to penicillin.

Ceclor®. Cefaclor is a cephalosporin antibiotic that has been found to be effective in the treatment of otitis media, but is expensive: a 10-day supply costs more than $20.

Gantrisin® is acetyl sulfisoxazole and is the choice of many doctors when giving patients a one-time daily dose over several months to prevent otitis media (see discussion below).

Augmentin® is a penicillin that contains clavulanic acid, which kills defensive enzymes created by certain bacteria.

Adverse Reactions to Antibiotics

An antibiotic that is given orally does not all rush to the site of the infection. If it did, there would be no side effects. Instead, the antibiotic is absorbed into the bloodstream and is circulated throughout the body. During its travels, the antibiotic interacts with many different microorganisms.

The most beneficial interaction occurs when the antibiotic reaches the site of an infection and kills bacteria. However, in many children who take antibiotics for middle ear infection, the antibiotic can alter the normal microbial "population" in the large intestine, causing diarrhea, the most common reaction to antibiotics used in the treatment of otitis media.

Parents should consider several general factors about antimicrobial treatment:

In very few instances are adverse reactions severe enough to warrant discontinuation of the medication.[1] However, check with a physician if there is any doubt about the severity of a side effect.

Long-term use of any particular antibiotic can result in the growth of bacteria resistant to that antibiotic. Therefore, some children will get an ear infection while on prophylactic use of antibiotics when a resistant bacteria grows and causes inflammation of the middle ear.

Prolonged use of some antibiotics can reduce the white blood cell count. A child taking certain sulfa-containing antibiotics for a long period of time should probably have the blood cell count checked regularly to make sure it has not fallen below normal levels.

The following are some common reactions to antibiotics regularly used in the treatment of otitis media:

Amoxicillin. Watery stools or diarrhea, if mild, are usually not a reason to discontinue. A nonallergic rash that may develop looks like isolated raised pink bumps on the skin. However, some children may have an allergic reaction to amoxicillin, most often manifested by smooth, raised welt-like lesions round, oval or irregular in shape that cover the body and itch and burn. If the child develops this rash, the antibiotic should be discontinued.[1]

Pediazole®. This drug should be stopped at the first appearance of skin rash or any other adverse reaction, according to the manufacturer. The most frequent side effects are abdominal cramping and discomfort. Infrequently, nausea, vomiting and diarrhea can occur.

Bactrim® and Septra®. Each of these drugs can cause nausea, vomiting, diarrhea and skin rashes. Most of these side effects should be mild and do not warrant discontinuation of the drug.[1] The manufacturer instructs that Bactrim® and Septra® are to be used in the treatment of acute otitis media "when in the judgment of the physician Bactrim® or Septra® offers some advantage over the use of other antimicrobial agents. To date, there are limited data on the safety of repeated use of Bactrim® or Septra® in children under two years of age. Septra® or Bactrim® is not indicated for prophylactic or prolonged administration in otitis media at any age."

Special precautions should be taken in using antibiotics combined with sulfisoxazole (Bactrim®, Septra®, Pediazole®, Gantrisin®):

- These medications should not be given to infants under two months of age.

- The antibiotics should be given with a lot of liquid, either water or milk, because the sulfa can be crystallized in the kidneys if it is not flushed out properly.

- In some children, these antibiotics can sensitize the skin to sun. Many pharmacists advise parents to keep children out of the sun while on these medications.

- These antibiotics can reduce white blood cell count.

- The "warnings" section included in the instructions provided with Bactrim®, Septra® and Pediazole® has been expanded at the request of the Food and Drug Administration (FDA). The FDA has received reports of adverse reactions, some of them fatal, in conjunction with these medications. Although fatalities are very rare, the FDA has alerted physicians to the frequency and potential severity of the reactions and advises them to monitor patients using these medications.[8]

Ceclor®. Besides diarrhea, an unusual reaction to Ceclor® is the eruption of red patches all over the body. This has usually occurred during or following a second course of therapy with the drug. These symptoms usually subside within a few days after the drug is stopped. Children who have had allergic reaction to penicillin may also be allergic to Ceclor®.[1]

GUIDELINES FOR TREATMENT
WITH ANTIBIOTICS ════════════

Acute Otitis Media

Those children with acute otitis media who are most vulnerable to serious illness and who should receive antibiotics immediately are newborn children with impaired immune systems or those who are undergoing chemotherapy for cancer.

With those exceptions, it may not be necessary to treat your child's acute ear infection with antibiotics. Studies have shown that, in many instances, acute symptoms of otitis media subside without treatment in 24 to 72 hours in 70 to 80 percent of children.[9,10,11] If you can relieve your child's ear pain with the use of topical anesthetic ear drops or non-aspirin liquid or tablet pain reliever or by applying heat to the affected ear, your child's symptoms may abate within 24 hours. If your child's pain persists for more than 24 hours, however, your physician may prescribe an antibiotic.

Middle Ear Fluid

Middle ear fluid commonly lingers for more than a month in up to 40 percent of children who have had an acute ear infection.[12] Parents should not consider antibiotics ineffective because a child still has fluid in the ear after a 10-day course of antimicrobial treatment. Most physicians will take a "wait and-see" approach for several months to let the fluid resolve spontaneously before considering another course of antibiotics.

Middle Ear Ventilation Disorder

Since mechanical factors, rather than infection, are primarily responsible for a retracted eardrum, most physicians would agree that antibiotics are ineffective and unnecessary in the treatment of this condition.

Frequently Occurring Acute Otitis Media

In recent years, physicians have begun using antibiotics in an attempt to prevent the frequent development of ear infections in children who are prone to otitis media. This preventive use of antibiotics is called prophylaxis or chemoprophylaxis. Prophylactic treatment includes giving a low dose of antibiotic on a daily basis over several months to help reduce episodes of otitis media.

Many doctors are enthusiastic about preventive use of antibiotics for children who suffer recurrent ear infections. Four separate reports suggest this treatment helps reduce recurrence of otitis media, although it will not eliminate the problem altogether.[13,14,15,16]

One study reported the findings that follow: (1) children under two years of age are most likely to benefit; (2) the parents must comply carefully with schedules for administering medication in order to ensure maximum benefits (dosages cannot be skipped); (3) children have less disease in the months after conclusion of the preventive regimen.[14]

Although some experts are enthusiastic about the possible benefits of this low-dose preventive management, no agreement has been reached as to the best antibiotic to use, though sulfa drugs and amoxicillin are most commonly prescribed.[17]

Drawbacks to prophylactic antimicrobial therapy include the following:

- Some children develop an acute infection while on the preventive medication. In this case, the physician will most likely change to a different antibiotic, prescribing a larger dose and more frequent administration than once daily.

- Prophylactic use of antibiotics has not been studied over a long period of time and has not been specifically approved by the U.S. Food and Drug Administration.[18]

- The white blood cell count of a child on long-term management with some antibiotics that contain sulfa can become abnormally and even dangerously low. If so, the antibiotic should be discontinued. Many doctors require children on prophylactic antibiotics to receive a blood cell count every eight weeks.

- Unpleasant side effects can occur, such as skin rash and upset stomach, although these have been noted infrequently.

- Recently, there have been reports of fungal infections in children who have been treated with prophylactic antibiotics.[19] Signs of fungal infections include fatigue, low-grade fever, lethargy.

In summary, the parent and doctor must weigh the advantages and disadvantages of using an antibiotic prophylactically. It may be an alternative to surgery and may decrease the number of times your child will have an ear infection over the winter months; however, the long-term effects are unknown, the medication may cause side effects, and the child may develop infections caused by other bacteria that are resistant to the antibiotic he is taking.

Persistent Middle Ear Fluid

Treatment of persistent middle ear fluid—more than 10 weeks in both ears—with antibiotics is a controversial subject among physicians. The major question is: what role does an antibiotic play in clearing middle ear fluid?

In the textbook *Pediatric Otolaryngology*, Charles D. Bluestone, M.D., and Jerome O. Klein, M.D., state that all children who have middle ear fluid, regardless of the stage, should receive an antibiotic if one has not been given in the last few months.[20] Their opinion is based on the fact that half the time middle ear fluid regularly contains some bacteria.[21] Since this bacteria is usually found to be the same as that in acute otitis media, the antibiotic chosen and the duration of treatment can be the same as that recommended for acute otitis media.

Another argument in favor of using antibiotics to help clear middle ear fluid is that the therapy is a last resort before removal of the fluid by myringotomy and possibly insertion of tubes in the ears.

Some doctors admit that they prescribe prophylactic antibiotics, even though the middle ear fluid really needs no treatment, because parents want something done rather than just waiting to see if the fluid will disappear.

Although some studies have shown that antimicrobial therapy hastens disappearance of middle ear fluid by killing bacteria,[22,23] conflicting opinions and results of other studies have left unanswered the question of whether this treatment can be successful.

How Many Days Should Antibiotics Be Taken?

Common length of treatment with antibiotics is 10 or 14 days. Often, parents are warned on the bottle's label: "Important: Finish all this medication unless otherwise instructed by physician." Many parents wonder why they should continue treatment for up to two weeks when the child improves in a day. Traditionally, a physician's answer has been that while the symptoms diminish rapidly, the antibiotic may need more time to clear the infection.

The origin of the 10-day course of therapy is unknown;[24,25] in fact, this length of therapy is being challenged by researchers today. Two studies in the last four years have shown that treatment for five days[26] and treatment for two days[27] is just as effective as treatment for 10 days.

More scientific studies are needed in order to determine the best length of time for antimicrobial treatment of otitis media. Shortened duration and decrease in quantity of antibiotics could save parents thousands of dollars—and many hours of inconvenience.

Why Doesn't the Antibiotic Work?

Antibiotics are ineffective against otitis media for three major reasons:

(1) The medicine is not administered according to the physician's or pharmacist's directions. For instance, a parent may ignore instructions on the bottle that direct her to give the medication along with food or with milk or water; or a parent may simply forget to give the child his or her dose.

Other reasons for noncompliance may be the parents' fear of side effects, lack of money to purchase the medication or hesitancy to give the medicine to an uncooperative child. Some children resist taking the medicine, and spit it out or regurgitate it. Even if the parents finally persuade the child to take some medicine, it is difficult to determine if the child swallowed the right dose. Consequently, parents are constantly thinking of games, ploys, bribes or threats to get their children to take the medicine. One mother said she disliked the antibiotic therapy. "During my child's first year, it seemed that I was constantly battling him to take this medicine," she said. "I resented having to struggle continually with him to give him the medicine."

Yet other parents hesitate to administer the medicine because they're not convinced the child really needs it. "I don't consider myself a fanatic opposed to antibiotics," said one mother, "but when my child had been on antibiotics continually for the first two years of his life, I began to question the treatment."

(2) The organisms causing the ear infection may be "resistant" to the medicine (as already described).

(3) The infection is caused by a microorganism other than bacteria, such as a virus. Antibiotics only kill bacteria and do not kill viruses.

Why Doesn't the Antibiotic Work?

- Medicine not administered correctly by parents
- Bacteria is resistant to antibiotic
- Ear infection is caused by virus, not bacteria

Can a Child Become Immune to Antibiotics? and How Much Is Too Much Antibiotic?

If a child has been on many different kinds of antibiotics for a long time, parents worry that: (1) the child will become immune to antibiotics; (2) the antibiotics will be harmful; or (3) the antibiotics will interfere with the body's natural defense mechanism. One mother expressed a common fear: "What happens if my child really becomes sick, like with meningitis or some other disease? Will he be so immune to antibiotics that nothing will work against the disease?"

Parents have a right to question why their child is on constant antimicrobial treatment. As discussed above, antibiotics are prescribed to eliminate bacteria during an acute ear infection. After the symptoms of the infection have passed, the remaining middle ear fluid usually does not contain large numbers of harmful bacteria. Therefore, once the full course of antibiotics has been taken for an acute ear infection, it probably is unnecessary to continue medication.

"Can my child become immune to antibiotics?" is one of the questions most commonly asked of pediatricians. The concept of a child becoming "immune" to an antibiotic is misleading. One cannot become immune to antibiotics; however, some bacteria can become resistant to certain antibiotics. The more an antibiotic is given, the greater the chance that the resistant bacteria will grow in larger numbers. This growth of resistant bacteria can cause a child to get an ear infection while on prophylactic antibiotics.

Do antibiotics kill "good" bacteria? If so, is this harmful to the child's health? Because antibiotics circulate through the blood system, they can interfere with or alter the numbers of bacteria normally found in the body. If the bacteria that normally live in the intestine are killed by an antibiotic, then diarrhea can develop. Also, if the bacteria that normally live in a girl's vagina are killed, a vaginal infection with yeast can develop. When bacteria that normally live in the mouth are killed, an oral infection with fungus (called thrush) can occur.

Can antibiotics discolor my child's teeth? The antibiotics commonly used to treat otitis media do not discolor teeth. Tetracycline—commonly given to children about 30 years ago—caused tooth discoloration in some instances.

Will antibiotics interfere with my child's own defense against infection? Some experts speculate that the continual use of antibiotics can prevent the body from building up its own defense mechanisms against bacteria (see further discussion in research section below).

RESEARCH IN ANTIMICROBIAL TREATMENT FOR OTITIS MEDIA ═══════════════

The most frequent types of studies involving antibiotics compare the efficacy of one antibiotic to another's. Most of these studies utilize two groups of children and treat them for otitis media with two different kinds of antibiotics. These studies examine such factors as: which medications cause fewer side effects; which are better absorbed; which kill bacteria faster; and which require fewer dosages.

Below are descriptions of the kinds of studies being conducted in the area of new antimicrobial treatments. Keep in mind that many studies are conducted before any new medication is used on a large scale. Additionally, some physicians are reluctant to use such medications until they see the results of several studies. The following examples give you an idea of the methodology of these studies.

Bacampicillin® was shown to be as effective as amoxicillin in the treatment of otitis media and easier to administer because Bacampicillin needed to be taken only twice a day.[6]

Another study showed that more children who received Ceclor® were free of effusion at 14 days after onset of therapy than children who received amoxicillin.[28]

Cyclacillin® was demonstrated to be better absorbed by the gastrointestinal tract than amoxicillin and, therefore, resulted in fewer side effects.[7]

Researchers found Augmentin® more effective than Ceclor® in resolving acute otitis media, but it caused more side effects, such as diaper rash and loose stools.[29]

CONTROVERSIES ABOUT ANTIMICROBIAL TREATMENT

With all due respect to the wonderful antimicrobials now available, more than merely the correct choice of one or a combination of antimicrobials is involved in the resolution of acute otitis media . . . we must look beyond the "drug-versus-bug" equation, keeping in mind that much more remains to be learned than we already know about the pathophysiology of this fascinating and common disease.[30]

Jack Paradise, M.D.
Children's Hospital,
Pittsburgh

Most physicians in the United States use antibiotics routinely as their first treatment of acute otitis media. Indeed many parents expect—and sometimes even demand—a prescription for antibiotics when their child has an ear infection. Numerous studies and researchers are now challenging the routine use of antibiotics in treating acute otitis media. Although serious disease associated with otitis media has declined in the last three decades, no study has shown that the decline is a result of the aggressive use of antibiotics.[31] Also, researchers are questioning whether the routine use of antibiotics is a contributing factor to frequently occurring acute otitis media and persistent middle ear fluid—conditions that were rare before the advent of antimicrobial therapy.[31,32]

Advantages of Antibiotic

- Kills bacteria, thereby helping to relieve pain and other symptoms of acute otitis media
- Can be used in children with persistent middle ear fluid or frequently occurring acute otitis media to promote resolution of fluid and reduce frequency of infections

Disadvantages of Antibiotic

- Possible side effects
- High cost, inconvenience
- Bacteria may become resistant to antibiotic

Jack L. Paradise, M.D., of the Children's Hospital of Pittsburgh suggests that: "Antimicrobial treatment should not be undertaken routinely but should be reserved for more severe or more complicated cases or for certain more vulnerable patients. Such an approach might allow for the better development of natural immunity in untreated subjects," he says, "and would certainly reduce the costs and complications of antimicrobial therapy."[33]

One factor not often discussed by experts, but which is a primary concern to parents, is the tremendous cost of antibiotics:

In 1977, the total cost for prescriptions purchased for treatment of otitis media was $88.6 million; that cost has risen over the last seven years to reach $156.8 million.[34]

It has been estimated that, of the 120 million prescriptions written for oral antibiotics annually in the United States, more than one fourth are used in the treatment of otitis media.[35]

In 1987, amoxicillin was prescribed in 39 percent of patient visits to office-based physicians where otitis media was diagnosed.[5] In 1985, Amoxil® (a specific brand of amocillin) was one of the top 20 best-selling prescription drugs in the United States.[36]

Studies examining the way in which antibiotics affect the course of otitis media are adding to the controversies:

- Antibiotics may change the chemical properties of bacteria and effusion so that fluid persists much longer than it would have without treatment of antibiotics.[32]

- Incomplete antibiotic therapy for an acute infection may allow bacteria to persist in the middle ear, causing continued irritation to the mucus. This prolonged irritation could produce inflammation that leads to persistent middle ear fluid.[37]

- Early antibiotic treatment of an initial ear infection may prevent the development of adequate immunity of the ear, particularly in children under two whose immune systems are being developed. Subsequent infection results in middle ear fluid due to incomplete development of immunity in the middle ear.[38]

- Should antibiotic therapy be used routinely in the treatment of acute otitis media? Should it be used immediately or can it be delayed?

- How long should an antibiotic be used: two days, five days, seven days, ten days?

- What antibiotic is most effective in treating acute otitis media?

- Is antimicrobial therapy effective in clearing middle ear effusion? And if so, which antibiotic is most effective?

Unfortunately, the answers to these perplexing questions are not yet available. As research continues, the answers will become available. In the meantime, physicians and parents must make decisions based on current theories and results of available studies.

QUESTIONS AND ANSWERS ━━━━━

Q: How do antibiotics relieve pain so quickly?

A: Bacteria cause pain as a result of inflammation and swelling in the middle ear. As the antibiotic kills bacteria, the inflammation and swelling subside.

Q: Why are there still bacteria in the middle ear fluid of a child who has been on antibiotics for 10 days?

A: No antibiotic is absolutely effective in totally eradicating all bacteria from the middle ear in all cases. The antibiotic is designed to kill most bacteria and then the body's defense mechanism must continue the work to cure the infection.

Q: If antibiotics are ineffective against the treatment of viral ear infections, how does a physician treat otitis media caused by a virus?

A: Ear infections that are caused by viruses are self-limited —that is, they almost always improve without medication. Viruses, which cause the common cold, are not cured by antibiotics.

Q: If I know that members of the family have had a history of allergy to penicillin or other antibiotics, could this mean that my child is also allergic to the same antibiotics?

A: Children of allergic parents have a greater risk of being allergic than children of nonallergic parents. In the case of antibiotics, a physician will not know if the child will be sensitive to a certain antibiotic unless the child is given the medication. Allergic parents should watch their children very carefully for any signs or symptoms of a reaction throughout treatment with antibiotics.

Q: My doctor always asks me to bring my child in for a "re-check" 10 days after the diagnosis of an ear infection to see if the antibiotic worked. Often, he switches to another antibiotic at that point. Why would he prescribe a second antibiotic when my child seems absolutely fine?

A: These questions, which are asked by many parents, are discussed fully on page 252. Briefly, here is a thumbnail answer:

Your doctor wants to see your child at the end of a 10-day course on an antibiotic to examine the ear and look for signs that would suggest that the infection is still active. However, if your child's ear pain and fever subsided within 24 hours after the antibiotic was initially given, and the symptoms of fever and pain did not recur, then the doctor can assume that the antibiotic was effective.

Although many doctors say that an antibiotic didn't "work" if they observe fluid in the ear after antibiotic has been given, the doctor cannot really tell if there are bacteria present without puncturing the eardrum and looking at a sample of fluid under a microscope, or culturing the bacterial growth. Since this is rarely done, the prescribing of a second antibiotic 10 days after giving a first antibiotic for an acute ear infection may be excessive therapy (see "Overdiagnosing and Misdiagnosing" on page 76).

The next time your doctor wants to give your child a second antibiotic right after completion of the first antibiotic, ask him to explain his rationale for the way he's managing your child's ear infections.

Q: **Why does my doctor sometimes prescribe an antibiotic that did not previously work for my child?**

A: Read carefully the section in this chapter on bacteria and "resistance" of organisms. The fact that fluid has lingered in your child's ear after an acute ear infection does not necessarily mean that the antibiotic was ineffective in killing bacteria. Further, the bacteria responsible for one ear infection may be different than the bacteria that caused a previous ear infection. Your doctor may choose to give for prophylactic therapy low dose amoxicillin even though your child had been taken off amoxicillin three months ago when the doctor found *fluid in your child's ear after completion of the 10 days on amoxicillin. In this example, the amoxicillin may have killed all the harmful bacteria in the ear when it was given for 10 days as treatment for the acute ear infection. You should not think that the amoxicillin "did not work" just because fluid remains in the ear after your child stops taking the antibiotic. Remember, it is probable that fluid will remain in a child's ear for more than a month after the acute infection has been treated effectively.*[12]

NOTES

1.   Peter G. Side Effects and Toxicity of Antimicrobial Agents and Development of Resistant Bacteria to Drugs. Pediatric Annals. 1984 May: 13(5): 370–376.
2.   Bluestone CD, Klein JO. "Otitis Media with Effusion, Atelectasis and Eustachian Tube Dysfunction" in Pediatric Otolaryngology Volume 1 (edited by CD Bluestone and SE Stool). 1983 WB Saunders Co.: 434.
3.   Clavulanic acid inhibits beta-lactamases. FDA Drug Bull. 1984 Dec;14(3):25.
4.   Schwartz, RH, Schwartz DM. Acute Otitis Media: Diagnosis and Drug Therapy. 1980: Drugs 19: 107–118.
5.   National Disease and Therapeutic Index 1987.
6.   Kim HK, Bluestone CD, et al. "Comparison of Bacampicillin and Amoxicillin for Acute Otitis Media" in Studies in Otitis Media, Pittsburgh Otitis Media Research Center Progress Report 1982 (SE Stool and CD Bluestone, editors). Annals Otol, Rhinol & Laryngol. 1983 Nov–Dec: Suppl 107:92(6:2):37–40.
7.   McLinn SE, Serlin S. Cyclacillin versus amoxicillin as treatment for acute otitis media. Pediatrics. 1982 Feb;71(2):196–99.
8.   Serious adverse reactions with sulfonamides. FDA Drug Bull. 1984 April; 14(1):5–6.
9.   van Buchem FI, Dunk JHM, van't Hof MA. Therapy of acute otitis media: Myringotomy, antibiotics or neither? Lancet 1981:883–887.
10.   Diamant M, Diamant B. Abuse and timing of use of antibiotics in acute otitis media. Arch otolaryngol 1974; 100:226–232.
11.   Fry J. Antibiotics in acute tonsillitis and acute otitis media. Br Med J 1958; 883–886.

12. Teele DW, Klein JO, Rossner B, et al. Epidemiology of Otitis Media in Children. Ann Otol Rhinol Laryngol 1980; 89 (suppl 68): 5–6.

13. Shurin PA. "Prevention of Otitis Media With Antimicrobial Drugs" in Otitis Media: Publication of the Second National Conference on Otitis Media (RJ Wiet and SW Coulthard, coeditors). 1979, Ross Laboratories, 1979: 67–69.

14. Klein JO. Antimicrobial Prophylaxis for Recurrent Acute Otitis Media. Pediatric Annals. 1984 May; 13(5): 398–403.

15. Schwartz RH, et al. Sulphanethoxazole Prophylaxes in the Otitis-prone Child. Arch Dis Child. 1982 Aug; 57 (8); 590–93.

16. Liston TE, et al. Sulfisoxazole Chemoprophylaxis for Frequent Otitis Media." Pediatrics 1983 April; 71(4) 524–30.

17. Shambaugh GE. "Complications of Otitis Media" in Otitis Media: Publication of the Second National Conference on Otitis Media (RJ Wiet and SW Coulthard, coeditors). 1979, Ross Laboratories: 48–50.

18. Grundfast KM. "Acute Otitis Media" in Current Emergency Therapy (Elich RF and Spyker DA, editors). Aspen. Rockville, MD. 1985: 921–925.

19. Crook WG. The Yeast Connection. Professional Books. Jackson, Tennessee. 1985: 209–211.

20. Bluestone CD, Klein JO. "Otitis Media with Effusion, Atelectasis and Eustachian Tube Dysfunction" in Pediatric Otolaryngology Volume 1 (edited by CD Bluestone and SE Stool). 1983 WB Saunders Co.: 460.

21. Lim DJ, DeMaria TF. "Bacteriology and Immunology." Laryngoscope. 1982 March: 92 (3): 278–286.

22. "Antibiotics Efficacious in Treating Otitis Media." Allergy Today, 1985 May: 2.

23. GB Healy. "Antimicrobial therapy of chronic otitis media with effusion." Int J Pediatr Otorhingolaryngol 1984 Oct; 8(1): 13–7.

24. Wright PF. Indication and Duration of Antimicrobial Agents for Acute Otitis Media. Pediatric Annals. 1984 May: 13 (5): 377–379.

25. Bluestone CD, Klein JO. "Otitis Media with Effusion, Atelectasis and Eustachian Tube Dysfunction" in Pediatric Otolaryngology Volume 1 (edited by CD Bluestone and SE Stool). 1983 WB Saunders Co.: 433.

26. Ingvarsson L; Lundgren K. "Penicillin treatment of acute otitis media in children. A study of the duration of treatment." Acta Otolaryngol (Stockh) 1982 Sep–Oct; 94 (3–4); 283–87.

27.   Meistrup-Larsen KI, et al. "Two versus seven days penicillin treatment for acute otitis media. A placebo controlled trial in children." Acta Otolaryngol (Stockh) 1983 Jul–Aug; 96 (1–2): 99–104.

28.   Giebink GS, Batalden PB, Ruso JN, Le Ct. "Cefaclor versus amoxicillin in the treatment of otitis media" in Recent Advances in Otitis Media (DB Lim, senior editor). 1984: B.C. Decker: 287–289.

29.   Odio CM, Kusmiesz H, Shelton S, Nelson JD. Comparative treatment trial of augmentin versus cefaclor for acute otitis media with effusion. Pediatrics 1985 May;75(5):819–26.

30.   Paradise JL. Inadequate Resolution of Acute Otitis Media Following Antimicrobial Therapy. Pediatric Annals. 1984 May;13(5): 382–390.

31.   Gates GA. "Management" in Recent Advances in Otitis Media With Effusion (Lim DJ, editor). Annals of Otology, Rhinol and Laryngol. 1985 Jan–Feb: Suppl 116, 94 (1;3) 27–30.

32.   Smyth G. Management of Otitis Media With Effusion: A Review. The American Journal of Otology. 1984 July; 5(5): 344–349.

33.   Paradise JL. "Otitis Media in Infants and Children." Pediatrics. 1980 May; 65 (5): 917–943.

34.   National Medical Expenditure Survey, Household Data: United States, 1977. National Center for Health Services Research.

35.   Bluestone CD. Otitis Media: Update 1984. Infectious Diseases. 1984 April: 14(4): 4.

36.   Information from a staff report prepared by the subcommittee on Health and the Environment of the Committee of Energy and Commerce of the U.S. House of Representatives (Henry A. Waxman, chairman): "Price Increases for Prescription Drugs and Related Information." July 15, 1985.

37.   Lim DJ, Schram JL, et al. Antibiotic Resistant Bacteria in Otitis Media with Effusion. Annals of Otol, Rhinol and Laryngol. 1980 May June. Suppl 68:89(3):278–280.

38.   Howie VM, Ploussard JH, Sloyer JL. "Natural History of Otitis Media" in Recent Advances in Otitis Media. Ann Otol Rhinol Laryngol. 1976; 85 Suppl: 25:18–19.

39.   Bluestone CD, workshop chairman. "Effects of Antimicrobial Agents on the Biological Activity of the Middle Ear With Otitis Media" in Studies in Otitis Media, Pittsburgh Otitis Media Research Center Progress Report 1982 (SE Stool and CD Bluestone, coeditors). Annals Otol, Rhinol and Laryngol. 1983 Nov–Dec; Suppl 107:92(Part 6, No. 2):48–50.

PART FIVE

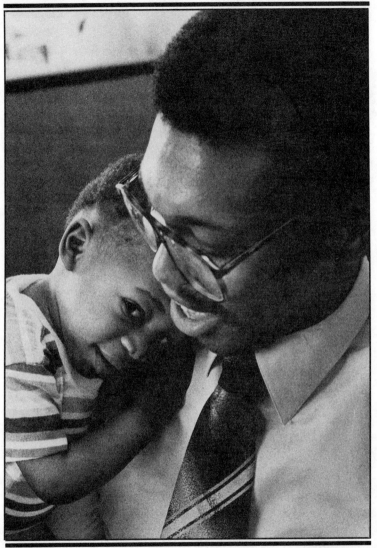

Ear
Tubes

CHAPTER ONE

Making the Decision to Insert Ear Tubes

Michael is 22 months old and has had five ear infections in the last three months. Though antibiotics rapidly diminish Michael's ear pain and fever, the fluid has remained in one or both ears for most of the past few months. Michael's parents, Anne and John, have noticed that he is having difficulty hearing. He says "What?" or "Huh?" all the time and wants the volume increased on the television or toy tape cassette player. His speech development has been a bit slow, and Anne has noticed that other children in the neighborhood speak more distinctly and have larger vocabularies. Because of all these factors, Michael's doctor suggested consultation with an ear specialist.

After an examination of Michael and discussion with the parents, the specialist recommended insertion of tympanostomy tubes to help reduce the frequency of ear infections. But John and Anne have many concerns. John says Michael is too young to have an operation and he's reluctant to agree to the surgery. Anne has heard and read negative reports about tympanostomy tubes. Both John and Anne are frightened about the prospect of Michael having general anesthesia. On the other hand, they realize Michael has been taking antibiotics almost constantly, without relief from the ear infections.

Anne and John find themselves in a situation many of their

153

counterparts are facing today: though their son is almost always ill with ear infections, has not been hearing well and should be speaking better, they remain unconvinced that insertion of tubes is really the answer. What should they do?

Unfortunately, there is no clear-cut answer. In this chapter, you'll learn how tympanostomy tubes work and when a doctor might recommend them. However, you'll find tympanostomy tubes are neither all good nor all bad, and that the criteria for insertion of tubes have never been clearly defined. This chapter explores the risks and benefits of tympanostomy tubes to help you make a decision about your child's treatment.

Tympanostomy Tubes Defined

The idea of placing a hollow tube into the eardrum to aerate the middle ear dates back to 1902, when Adam Politzer described a procedure for puncturing the eardrum and inserting a tube made of rubber. Although Dr. Politzer's early attempt to use the tympanostomy tube in treatment of otitis media met with some success, the procedure was not widely accepted because sterile techniques had not been perfected and the rubber tubes probably became a site for infection. Also, making an opening in the eardrum and inserting a small tube was rather difficult for the ear surgeon because the surgical microscope had yet to be invented and methods for administering general anesthesia had not been perfected.

In 1954, Beverly Armstrong reported success in management of otitis media with insertion into the eardrum of tiny hollow tubes made of synthetic, inert and nonreactive materials. The tubes were inserted under sterile conditions and were not rejected by the body. Since Dr. Armstrong reported his work to the American Academy of Otolaryngology and Ophthalmology, the use of tympanostomy tubes in treatment of otitis media has become widespread.

Tympanostomy tubes today are commonly referred to as ventilation tubes or just "tubes." Tympanostomy is derived from Greek and Latin: "tympano" is the Greek word for drum and "ostum" is the Latin word for door, entrance or mouth. Therefore, tympanostomy means an entrance in the drum; in this case, the eardrum. Tympanostomy tubes are also called by other names, such as grommets (which is a particular type of tube); drain tubes or P.E. (pressure equalization) tubes.

How Tubes Work

There is nothing magical or sophisticated about the way in which tympanostomy tubes work. Quite simply, a tympanostomy tube is merely a tiny hollow tube about the size of this dot "@" through which air can pass. To understand how a tympanostomy tube works, think of it as a temporary artificial eustachian tube. That is, the tympanostomy tube maintains an opening in a child's eardrum to allow air to enter the middle ear.

Most parents think a tympanostomy tube's primary purpose is to drain fluid from the middle ear. Although that is one

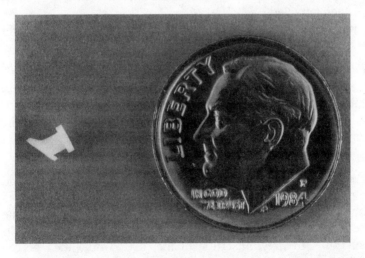

A tube can be as small as a fingertip. Above, a tube is photographed next to a dime to show children and parents how small it actually is. *(Photo by Jerry A. McCoy)*

function of the tube, it's primary function is to ventilate the middle ear by providing a hole in the eardrum for a defined length of time. If doctors could make a hole in a child's eardrum that would stay open for one or two years while the eustachian tube matures, tympanostomy tubes would be unnecessary.

When Tubes May Be Needed

By aerating and draining the middle ear, tympanostomy tubes can diminish the frequency of acute middle ear infections and prevent persistent middle ear fluid. Also, tympanostomy tubes can alleviate discomfort and improve hearing in children who have chronic negative middle ear pressure. Finally, insertion of a tympanostomy tube in a retracted eardrum can correct structural changes that have occurred and prevent the destruction of the middle ear bones or development of cholesteatoma (see page 90) that might occur if the eardrum were to become further retracted.

Here's a summary of the conditions for which a doctor might advise insertion of tympanostomy tubes:

Frequently occurring acute otitis media. A child who suffers recurrent ear infections (more than four ear infections in each of two consecutive seasons) despite prophylactic antimicrobial treatment may be a candidate for tubes. While the tubes will not "cure" the child of recurrent infections, they may reduce the frequency.

Persistent middle ear fluid. An ear surgeon may recommend removal of fluid and insertion of tubes in a child who has had fluid in both ears for more than 10 weeks, who has had some hearing loss and who has not responded to appropriate antimicrobial therapy. Insertion of the tubes would then be expected to restore hearing to normal (provided there is no sensorineural hearing loss, see Part Six). If the fluid is in only one ear, the doctor may remove the fluid (myringotomy) as an office procedure before a decision is made to insert a tube in the eardrum.

Middle ear ventilation disorder. When a child has poor eustachian tube function which results in a severely retracted eardrum that rests on the incus or stapes bone, then insertion of a tympanostomy tube in the eardrum can improve aeration of the middle ear and allow the eardrum to return to a normal position. This can also possibly prevent development of a cholesteatoma (see page 90). Sometimes, children with borderline adequate eustachian tube function will complain of vague ear discomfort, "popping" in the ears, or even mild hearing loss. Tubes can help equalize pressure and alleviate these symptoms.

Ear Tubes

Short-term benefits of tubes

- Restores hearing
- Prevents structural damage to eardrum

Long-term benefits of tubes

- May reverse chronic middle ear problem so that reinsertion is not necessary

Disadvantages of tubes

- Swimmers have to wear ear plugs
- Possible discharge from ears
- Tubes may fall out too early
- Damage to eardrum such as scarring, permanent hole
- Researchers are unaware of possible long-term damage

MAKING THE DECISION
TO INSERT TUBES

If your primary care physician believes tubes are a treatment option for your child, he will refer you to an ENT specialist for a final determination. How will you and the specialist arrive at your decision? The specialist's decision regarding insertion of tubes should take into consideration not only the child's physical ear condition and history, but the degree to which it is interfering with his daily routine and overall development.

Certain assumptions can be kept during the decision-making process: more often than not, middle ear fluid resolves without treatment (unless it is persistent, as defined above); as the child matures, the likelihood of spontaneous resolution increases; and, longer fluid-free periods mean the condition may clear up more quickly in the future.[1]

The decision to have tympanostomy tubes inserted in a child's ears is never easily made—either by a doctor or parents. Before making that decision, consider many of the factors discussed below:

Indications. When doctors consider the necessity of a surgical procedure, they talk about "indications" for surgery. By this, they mean there are accepted criteria for needing a certain type of operation. The indications, or criteria, usually include a generally accepted set of signs and symptoms, as well as laboratory, X-ray and other tests. For example, an individual is "indicated" for an appendectomy if he has acute onset of pain in the right lower portion of the abdomen, tenderness to pressure in the same area, fever, and an elevated white blood cell count.

Unfortunately, the indications for insertion of tympanostomy tubes have never been so clearly defined. However, this lack of well-defined indications for insertion of tympanostomy tubes should not give a physician an excuse to take a dogmatic or simplistic approach to the issue. Sometimes, this rigid approach can lead to excessive prescribing of antibiotics and procrastination in referring the child to an ENT specialist, which can make what was a relatively simple middle ear problem into a more complex condition.

Discussion of Indications. If your child has one or more of the conditions listed in the previous section, and neither antimicrobial therapy or a period of watchful waiting has led to improvement, then tympanostomy tubes may be helpful and beneficial; conversely, if your child has none of the conditions, his ear problems may not be serious enough to warrant the procedure. Remember, tubes are not a life-saving device; rather, they help reduce the frequency of ear infections and restore and preserve normal hearing. So, the decision does not have to be made immediately. Parents should take their time, discuss alternatives with the doctor, and learn about the procedure before reaching a decision.

When a doctor recommends that tubes be inserted, make him define the condition that warrants the procedure. Even if your child has had very frequent ear infections, if the infections are successfully treated with antibiotics and the eardrums return to normal soon after each infection, then tubes may not be needed. Also, prophylactic antibiotic therapy (see Part Four) should be attempted to help reduce the frequency of ear infections before a decision is made to insert tubes.

On the other hand, if your child has had only a few symptomatic acute ear infections, but has had persistent middle ear fluid in one or both ears, then its impact on hearing should be a major factor in making a decision about tubes. Monitoring of the hearing with hearing tests may help indicate whether or not tubes are needed. Remember that fluid can be removed from a child's ears without insertion of a tube (see Part Three, on myringotomy). Therefore, if your child's main problem is persistent fluid in one or both ears and has caused significant hearing loss, you should talk with the ear doctor about removal of fluid from the ears before making the decision that tubes are necessary.

Children with cleft palate, Down syndrome or some other

congenital or inherited disorder may have special reasons for insertion of tubes. For example, since children with cleft palate are born with an absent or deficient muscle to open the eustachian tube, they will have chronic middle ear problems throughout the childhood years.[2] Tympanostomy tubes are very helpful in alleviating chronic ear infections and middle ear fluid in such children.

Children with Down syndrome also tend to have poor eustachian tube function and chronic middle ear effusion, but extremely small canals can be a part of the syndrome, which can make the insertion of tubes quite difficult (or impossible). However, many Down syndrome children have benefitted greatly from them.

If your child has a condition (such as dwarfism, immotile cilia syndrome, mucopolysaccharide disorder) which interferes with normal middle ear function, a doctor may recommend insertion of tympanostomy tubes. Ask the doctor to explain how middle ear function is impaired and why tympanostomy tubes will be helpful.

Age. Can a child be too young or too old for insertion of tympanostomy tubes? Tubes can be inserted at any time during childhood, but are most helpful to children between the ages of 1 and 4 when ear infections occur frequently.

Although tubes sometimes need to be inserted in infant's ears, such a child's infections can be controlled with medication and an occasional myringotomy. Some doctors insert the tubes in infants without anesthesia as an office procedure. General anesthesia is safe for infants—as long as it's administered by a skilled anesthesiologist who has experience working with babies.

Unless a child has allergies or some other abnormal condition, infections usually will decrease when the child is four; the older the child gets, the more likely he will "outgrow" his ear infections. Therefore, if your three-and one-half-year-old has had frequent acute ear infections and a doctor recommends insertion of tympanostomy tubes, you might want to wait three to six months before making a final decision to see if the frequent episodes of otitis media diminish, especially if spring or summer is approaching.

Season. In temperate climates with distinct seasonal changes, acute otitis media occurs more frequently during the autumn and winter than during the spring and summer. Ear infections often accompany upper respiratory infections, which are more prevalent during autumn and winter. Therefore, children can benefit most from tympanostomy tubes that are in the eardrums and functional during cool-weather seasons. If tubes are inserted in the spring after your child has experienced a winter of multiple ear infections, you will never really know if the tubes were responsible for a reduction of ear infections, or if the ear infections decreased because of warm weather.

There are two additional reasons for waiting until after the summer to insert tympanostomy tubes. First, most doctors recommend that children with tubes should not get water in their ear canals when swimming. This can be difficult with young children who cannot understand the importance of keeping water out of the ears. If insertion can be delayed until after the summer, then a child will be free to enjoy swimming and water sports without ear protection.

Second, for the school age child who has had frequent episodes of otitis media and persistent middle ear fluid, sustained normal hearing is most important during the school year. If tubes are inserted during the springtime, then they may become blocked or extruded from the eardrum at some time during the middle of the school year when auditory acuity is of paramount importance. On the other hand, if tubes are inserted in the late summer or early autumn, then they will probably function properly and assure normal hearing throughout the entire school year.

Speech and language delays. Any child with frequent ear infections and/or persistent middle ear fluid who is showing signs of delayed speech and language development should be considered a candidate for insertion of tubes. The greater the degree of hearing loss and impairment of speech development, the more likely that the child will benefit from tubes. Although the relationship between otitis media and delayed speech development is yet to be scientifically proven (see Part Six), common sense should tell you that a young child with significant hearing impairment from longstanding fluid in both ears is likely to have more trouble with speech development than a child of comparable age with normal hearing.

COMPLICATIONS AND PROBLEMS WITH TUBES

Perforated Eardrum (Hole in the Eardrum). The major complication that can occur after a tympanostomy tube has been inserted is permanent perforation at the site where the tube is placed in the eardrum. When this occurs, surgical patching or grafting may be necessary to repair the hole. However, since the purpose of a tympanostomy tube is to keep open a hole in the eardrum, a small hole is not necessarily a problem. In fact, hearing can be entirely normal in an ear with a small hole in the eardrum. The doctor may advise waiting until the child is eight before recommending surgical repair of a small hole because the doctor wants the child's body to mature and develop better eustachian tube function before the procedure. Ideally, once the hole in the eardrum is closed, the child's eustachian tube must provide transfer of air into the middle ear without artificial help.

Early Extrusion. The length of time that a tympanostomy tube stays in the eardrum varies according to the design of the tube. Most tubes are designed to remain in a child's eardrum from six months to two years. If your child's tube comes out of the eardrum within eight weeks after insertion, this is a complication. Early extrusion usually means there was a technical problem with the way in which the tube was inserted. The doctor may be able to reinsert the tube in his office instead of returning to the operating room.

Failure to Extrude. Sometimes, a tube does not spontaneously extrude from the eardrum. If a tube that was not intended to remain in a child's eardrum permanently has not come out within two years, then it may have to be removed by the ear specialist. Doctors are usually reluctant to leave tubes in for more than two years because risk of permanent perforation increases with time in the eardrum. Soft silicone tubes such as the "T-tube" can usually be removed as an office procedure. Removal of harder tubes such as the fluoroplastic grommet tubes may require general anesthesia. If your child does require general anesthesia for removal of a tube from the ear, then the doctor may want to patch the hole just to help avoid the possibility he will be left with a permanent perforation at the site.

Occluded (Plugged) Tube. The hollow center of the tube is called the "lumen" and the lumen must remain open in order for air to pass through the tube. If the lumen becomes occluded (plugged) by ear wax or dried middle ear fluid, then the tube is of no benefit to the child even though it's in proper position. When a tube becomes occluded and fails to act as a conduit for air, then your child can begin to have the frequent ear infections and persistent middle ear fluid that occurred before the tube was inserted.

Your primary care doctor usually can determine if a tube lumen has become plugged by examining the ear with an otoscope. A tympanogram can also provide information that will help confirm that a tube lumen has become occluded. If occlusion has occurred, instillation of antibiotic/steriod ear drops into the ear canal may unplug the tube, or, an ear surgeon may be able to remove the debris using a microscope and tiny instruments.

Even if all attempts fail to unplug a blocked tympanostomy tube, the tube does not necessarily have to be removed, even though your child will not benefit from having it. Usually, the ear doctor will tell you that your child may get ear infections and/or fluid in the ear with the blocked tube, but he probably will advise waiting until the tube spontaneously extrudes rather than surgically removing the non-functioning tube, because removal would be painful and might tear the eardrum. Further, it is best for the tube to come out by itself gradually so that the eardrum can slowly heal as it comes out.

Drainage Through the Tube. Green, yellow or amber liquid can drain through the tube into the ear canal and then be seen dripping from the outer ear. Usually, this occurs within one or two days after the appearance of typical cold symptoms such as watery eyes, runny nose, cough and nasal congestion.

The ear drainage indicates an excessive amount of mucus within the middle ear which is draining through the tube. Excessive mucus production occurs as a response to infection. When your child has an upper respiratory infection (common cold), large amounts of mucus are produced in the nose, sinuses and in the middle ear. If your child seems to have an ordinary cold without other worrisome symptoms such as fever and you notice one or both ears are beginning to drain yellowish, sticky fluid (mucus), you might wait two or three days to see if the ear drainage subsides before going to a doctor. Also, you might discuss with the ear doctor the advisability of instilling eardrops to liquify the sticky mucus and help prevent the tympanostomy tubes from becoming blocked by dried mucus.

As a parent, you should not become alarmed by drainage from your child's ears after tympanostomy tubes have been inserted, since the drainage is not necessarily bad. After all, if the tubes were not in the eardrums, then the infected mucus would have been confined in the middle ear space, causing bulging of the eardrum and pain. Even though the primary purpose of a tympanostomy tube is to ventilate rather than drain the middle ear, a secondary benefit is its ability to provide an easy exit route for infected mucus.

However, if your child has had tubes inserted and then has nearly constant drainage from one or both ears without associated symptoms of an upper respiratory infection, something is wrong. Just as infected mucus can exit the middle ear through a tympanostomy tube, some doctors believe that harmful bacteria can enter the middle ear through a tube. This can occur if your child goes swimming and water containing harmful bacteria or viruses fills the ear canal, then travels through the tube into the middle ear. If this happens, then your doctor may advise instilling antibiotic ear drops in the ear canal and prescribe an oral antibiotic.

Some doctors believe that harmful organisms can enter the middle ear through the opening in a tympanostomy tube, even if a child avoids swimming. Therefore, hygiene is important. The ear canals and outer ears should be kept clean. Dirt, sand, or other unclean particles in the ear canal can lead to middle ear infection and ear drainage.

Regardless of the cause, ear drainage in a child with tympanostomy tubes usually stops within two or three days without any treatment, or soon after the doctor provides some type of treatment. Sometimes, however, children with allergies can have chronic drainage despite all types of treatment because the lining of the middle ear becomes swollen and can chronically weep a watery fluid through the tube into the ear canal. If your child is tested for, and then proved to have allergies, then an attempt will be made to control the allergies before deciding to remove tympanostomy tubes.

Rarely, a child with tympanostomy tubes can have chronic drainage from one or both ears with no identifiable cause. Although some doctors and parents talk of these children as being "allergic" to the tubes or "rejecting" the tubes, these concepts are probably not accurate in most instances. Nonetheless, if chronic drainage continues, and no cause can be found, the tubes may have to be removed.

Malposition of the Tube. After a tube has been in the eardrum for several months, the tube can turn as the eardrum grows. Usually, this does not interfere with function of the tube, but the doctor may not be able to view the end of the tube's lumen. If your doctor cannot see into the hollow portion of the tube, he may request tympanometry to check if the tube's lumen is open. Very rarely, the tube can become turned in such a way that it can actually be trapped in the middle ear. If this happens, your ear doctor should be able to look through the eardrum and see the tube lying in the middle ear. The ear doctor must remove a tube trapped in the middle ear after your child has been fully anesthetized by making an opening in the eardrum, and then grasping and removing the tube.

Scarring and Damage to the Eardrum. Whenever an incision is made in any part of the body, the healing process can lead to formation of a scar. Therefore, a scar can develop in the eardrum at the site where a tube had been. The scar can be thin and superficial or thick and hard. Although a doctor may be able to see a "scar" on the eardrum, most of the scars that are caused by insertion of a tympanostomy tube are small and do not interfere at all with hearing. However, an entire portion of an eardrum can become opaque and thickened if the body reacts to insertion of a tube by producing and depositing a substance called hyaline at the site where a tube has been in the eardrum. When this happens, the dense scar that can involve a portion of the eardrum is called a tympanosclerotic plaque. Even though the white plaque makes the eardrum look very abnormal, it usually does not interfere significantly with hearing.

NOTES ▬▬▬▬▬▬▬▬▬▬▬▬▬▬▬

1.   Paradise JL. On Tympanostomy Tubes: Rationale, Results, Reservations and Recommendations. Pediatrics. 1977 July: 60(1):86–90.
2.   Curtis AW, Clemis JD. "Middle Ear Effusions: Part 1—Pathophysiology." The Journal of Continuing Education in O.R.L. and Allergy. 1979 May:13–25.

Inserting
Ear Tubes

How Tubes Are Inserted

A tympanostomy tube is placed in an incision made in the eardrum. The ear canal is usually cleaned before the tube is inserted and the procedure is almost always done under a microscope. After the incision is made, the physician aspirates any fluid in the middle ear before inserting the tube. Tubes can be inserted without anesthesia, with local anesthesia or with general anesthesia (discussed below).

A tube is not sutured to the eardrum, but remains fixed in the eardrum the same way a button stays after being pushed through a button hole. Unless a tube becomes malpositioned or touches the ear canal wall, your child cannot feel or poke the tube.

Different Kinds of Tubes

An ever-growing assortment of sizes and shapes of tympanostomy tubes has become available during the past several years. Each tube is designed for a different purpose: a short-term tube usually stays in for less than a year and has a small hole; long-term tubes can remain for several years and may have to be surgically removed.

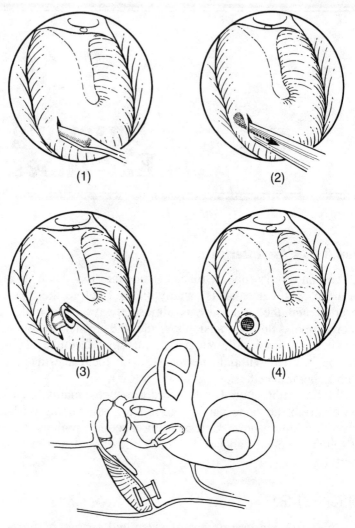

(1)   (2)   (3)   (4)

The insertion of a tympanostomy tube is preceded by a myrin-gotomy (an incision of the eardrum). Second, fluid is aspirated from the middle ear. Third, the tube is placed into the incision of the eardrum with a small pair of tweezers. The bottom drawing shows the tube's position in the eardrum so that one side is in the middle ear and the other is in the outer ear.

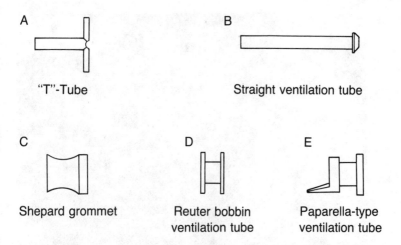

A "T"-Tube

B Straight ventilation tube

C Shepard grommet

D Reuter bobbin ventilation tube

E Paparella-type ventilation tube

Tubes are made of silicone rubber, stainless steel, fluoro-plastic or polyethylene and are available in different colors. Some long-term tubes have a larger inner flange (the part of the tube that rests on the inside of the eardrum) than short-term tubes. Others "spring back" to their original size after being compressed through the incision, or have tabs or wire attached to them so that the physician can pull them out easily. Still others are blue so the physician can see them easily, and some can be rotated after insertion to lock in place, or flap open like an umbrella when placed in the eardrum.

METHODS FOR INSERTION

In the Doctor's Office

Many children over age 5 (and some aged 3–5) who are co-operative and not frightened of physicians can hold still long enough so that the physician can insert tubes with only a local anesthetic. In this process, called iontophoresis, the ear canal is filled with a solution through which an electrical current is passed for 10 minutes. The child must lie still for the procedure which deadens the eardrum (see page 122 for discussion of iontophoresis).

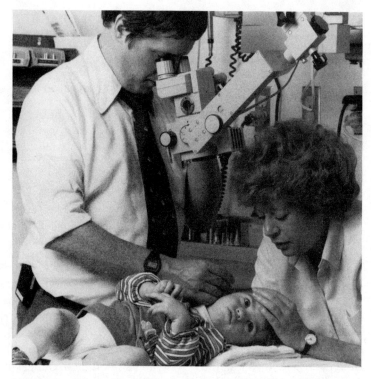

An otomicroscope is used by the surgeon to insert tympanostomy tubes. *(Photo by Donna K. Cantor)*

In children under 12 months, some physicians will insert tubes without any anesthesia in their office by having the child's head and body restrained. Although the procedure is painful, it is very quick and apparently tolerated without much after-effect in most babies.

In the Operating Room

Most often, tympanostomy tube insertion is performed on an outpatient basis in the hospital or an outpatient surgical center. The procedure takes only 30 minutes; however, because the child is given general anesthesia, he must stay in the hospital for several hours after surgery to make sure there are no ill effects from the anesthesia.

Preparing for Surgery in the Hospital

The child who is prepared for a trip to the operating room will suffer less anxiety than one who enters the hospital or surgical center without any forewarning. One mother described her son's reaction:

> *They opened the doors to the operating room. The whole room was white, and the doctor that Jerome knew so well was all covered in green. Jerome cried so loud that we could hear him from the waiting room. Then all of a sudden there was this silence . . .*

On the other hand, a hospital experience can be a very positive and even exciting experience for a child. One four-year-old didn't take off his hospital identification bracelet for weeks after the surgery. The boy's mother said he took off the bracelet only once when they returned to the hospital for a checkup, so that they wouldn't put him back in the hospital, she recalled.

Turning the hospital experience into a positive one can be accomplished by parents who prepare both themselves and their child by talking over fears, becoming familiar with hospital procedures, reading books about hospital experiences and visiting the hospital before the day of surgery.

The Parents' Preparation

Even though insertion of tubes is a common surgery that is done in thousands of children with little risk, parents rightfully have many fears about general anesthesia and surgery. Parents should not ignore or be ashamed of these fears. Any type of surgery in a loved one, especially a child, is going to provoke feelings of fear, guilt and anxiety. Since a parent's feelings about the experience often affect a child's perspective, it's important for parents to face these fears.

Although parents will not be able to erase all their fears, talking them over with a spouse, relatives and friends may help put the parent more at ease. The parents may ask themselves: How do I feel about my child going into the hospital? Am I afraid of a surgical mistake, or that my child will be harmed by the anesthesia? Will I be strong enough for my child when he is taken away to the operating room? Once aware of his or her own fears and feelings, it's easier for a parent to deal with the child's feelings.

It's helpful to find out as much about the experience as possible: talk to friends who have gone through the procedure and ask the ENT specialist about surgical risks and how the anesthesia is administered.

Finally, find out about the specifics of the hospital procedure, using the checklist provided.

Checklist for Preparing for Surgery in Hospital

_____ Date and time of surgery

_____ When are blood and urine tests taken?

_____ What events could mean surgery is postponed?

_____ No food or drink after midnight of the day of surgery

_____ When should child be at hospital?

_____ How long is the wait before and after surgery?

_____ How long does surgery last?

_____ Can parents remain with child while child is being anesthetized?

_____ Can parents be with child when she awakens in recovery room?

Preparing the Child

Children develop fears about hospitals and doctors as one way of coping with a strange and frightening experience. Children faced with separation from their parents and a potentially painful experience will try to "reason out" the event. Children over age three or four may think they are being punished for something they did wrong; younger children who hear words during snatches of conversations may take those words literally: "tubes" may mean garden hoses to them; "drawing blood" may mean taking all the blood out of their body; "being put to sleep" may mean that they'll wake up during the operation.

These fears may surface only in a chance remark that a parent may not even notice unless she is listening closely during the child's play. For instance, the child may put a doll in her "hospital bed." "Here's a tube that I'm going to put in your head," the little girl might say to the doll. "Now just go to sleep and try not to wake up while I put it in your ear." These misconceptions and fears can be somewhat alleviated if parents ask their children to describe what they think is going to happen to them. Some questions you can ask to prod your older (over age four) child are: "Do you know what's going to happen in the hospital? Why is it going to happen?" Start talking about the surgery about a week before the scheduled date to give the child time to think it over and ask questions.

What about the younger child? For the child aged 2 to 4, wait until a couple of days before the surgery since these children have a poor sense of time. They probably will respond best to a book, a tour of the hospital and some "play acting" of doctor and patient.

The baby or toddler, particularly between 9 and 18 months, will have the hardest time separating from her parents. Find out if you can stay with your child during the administration of anesthesia and if you can be with her when she wakes up in the recovery room.

How should parents respond to the fears of a child who is

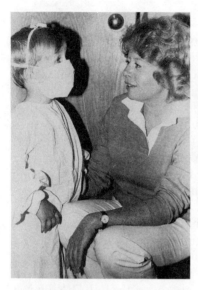

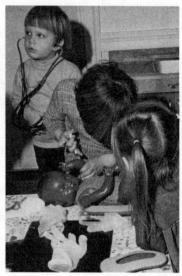

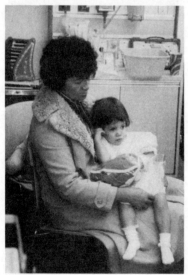

These photographs show children preparing for a day in surgery. Above, a child tries on a hospital gown and mask—the very clothing that his physician will wear on the day of surgery. At right, children play with stethoscopes and other examining instruments and practice being "doctors" on their doll "patients." Below, a mother and child in the waiting room before surgery. *(Photos courtesy of the Association for the Care of Children's Health)*

going to have tubes inserted in her ears? First, make sure the child knows how small the tubes really are. Many children may believe that "tubes" are as large as a garden hose. Ask the ENT specialist to show the child a real tube before surgery. Second, tell the child the doctor is going to put a "mask" on her face, or will give her an injection to put her to sleep and keep her from feeling the operation. Many children fear they'll awaken and feel pain during the operation.

For children over age one, books may help to alleviate fears and initiate discussion about upcoming surgery. The following books are recommended for children before entering the hospital. Other books may be recommended by your local librarian, or the librarian at the hospital.

Younger children: *Curious George Goes to the Hospital,* by Margaret Rey, Houghton Mifflin, 1966; *Miffy in the Hospital,* by Dick Bruna, Price Stern, 1982.

Preschoolers: *Why Am I Going to the Hospital?* by Claire Ciliotta and Carole Livingston, Lyle Stuart Inc., 1981; *A Surprise for Krissy,* by Sandra Ziegler, Child's World, 1976; *Elizabeth Gets Well,* by A. Weber, Crowell, 1970.

Preschoolers: *Koko Bear's Big Earache* by Vicki Lansky, Bantam, 1987; *Why Am I going to the Hospital?* by Claire Ciliotta and Carole Livingston, Lyle Stuart Inc., 1981; *A Surprise for Krissy,* by Sandra Ziegler, Child's World, 1976; *Elizabeth Gets Well,* by A. Weber, Crowell, 1970.

Kindergarten and older: *Hospital Roadmap: A Book to Help Explain the Hospital Experience to Young Children,* by Ingrid Glatz Elliott, Resources for Children, 1984; *Hospital Book,* by James Howe, Crown Publishers Inc., 1981; *Operation,* by Penny Anderson, Child's World, 1979.

For both parents and children: *Hospital Story: An Open Family Book for Parents and Children Together,* by Sarah Bonnett Stein, Walker and Company, 1984.

Finally, the child age two to four can be taken to the hospital for a special tour of the operating room and recovery room and for a discussion of hospital procedures. Some hospitals sponsor puppet shows during these tours, and the children are often allowed to try on the hospital gowns and masks.

The parent who wants more information about preparing the child for a hospital experience can send for *A Child Goes to the Hospital,* available for 75 cents from the Association

for the Care of Children's Health (ACCH), 3615 Wisconsin
Ave. NW, Washington, D.C., 20016; (202) 244-1801.

THE DAY OF SURGERY

Postponement of Surgery

Insertion of tympanostomy tubes is "elective" surgery—that
is, it is not performed to save a life and can be scheduled when
the child is healthy and at a convenient time for the parents.
If, on the day of surgery, the surgeon or anesthesiologist determines the child is not healthy, surgery may be postponed.
Some of the reasons for this include:

Noncompliance with instructions. It is important to follow
the hospital's instructions about fasting before surgery. A child
must have an empty stomach when given an anesthetic to
reduce the danger of vomiting and inhaling stomach contents
into the lungs while asleep. If these instructions are not followed, the surgery will be postponed. Generally, children are
not allowed solid food after midnight on the day of surgery.
Some hospitals allow children under one year of age to have
a small amount of water up to four hours before surgery.

Upper respiratory infection.   If the child has a cold, the
anesthesiologist may decide to postpone surgery because the
mucus could interfere with breathing or may get trapped in
the windpipe and go into the lungs.

Ear infection.   If the child has an infection, the surgeon may
postpone surgery until the eardrum has returned to normal.

Entering the Hospital for Surgery

Surgery takes place on an outpatient basis in a hospital or free-
standing or outpatient surgical center. That means the child is
admitted to the hospital a few hours prior to surgery and is
discharged a few hours after the general anesthesia wears off.

For example, if the surgery takes place in the morning, the child is usually home by 3 p.m. that same day.

On the morning of surgery, or a few days before, the child may be asked to give blood and urine samples. Many states and hospitals require these screening tests for surgical patients.

Undergoing General Anesthesia

Many parents are more concerned about anesthesia than about the surgery itself. Severe complications associated with anesthesia during insertion of ear tubes are extremely rare. Because an anesthesiologist is keenly aware that a child's body can react unexpectedly to anesthesia, he monitors the child's heart rate, blood pressure, temperature and electro-cardiogram continously; in fact, two anesthesiologists stay with the child while she is asleep. Because of the careful monitoring, any problems can be quickly detected and treated promptly. Another reason that complications are so rare is that the child is anesthesized for less than 30 minutes, since surgery lasts only about 10 minutes.

Children under age 2 and children who have such problems as heart disease or asthma, or any chronic illness will be taken to the operating room immediately after separation from parents for anesthesia. These children are most at risk for reactions and are monitored from the very beginning of induction of anesthesia. However, in some hospitals, generally healthy children over age 2 can be accompanied by their parents to an "induction" room where the parents can remain with the child until she falls asleep.

Most hospitals administer the anesthesia—a combination of halothane, nitrous oxide (laughing gas) and oxygen—through a mask. The children breathe the gas until they fall asleep. The gas has been described as smelling like strong mint or nail polish remover.

In the induction room, however, an anesthesiologist may give the child an injection while his parents are there before administering the anesthesia with a mask. The anesthesiologist injects the child if he suspects she will be uncooperative in using the mask or will be extremely frightened of the mask, or if the parents ask for the injection.

After surgery, the child breathes pure oxygen through the mask until she begins to wake up. She is then taken to a recovery room, where her condition continues to be monitored until she is fully awake. In many hospitals, the parents are allowed in the recovery room. Often the child acts groggy when the parents first see her, but most recover quickly.

Some children feel nauseous, dizzy, or may vomit from the anesthesia. Therefore, your child will be kept in the waiting room for several hours until she is awake, alert and able to drink fluids without vomiting.

After the Surgery — "She's a New Child!"

Most children exhibit no ill effects after surgery. In fact, many parents report their child is up and running around within an hour after awakening from the anesthesia. Some describe their child as a "new person" after surgery. If the child is old enough to talk, she may tell you she can hear sounds that she hadn't been able to hear before. One mother said her daughter sang all the way home because she was so thrilled to hear the sound of her voice. When she got home, the daughter was drinking soda and suddenly stopped to listen to the fizzle. "Do you hear that funny noise?" she asked.

Other parents remark that their children are happier because the discomfort associated with middle ear fluid disappears after insertion of tubes. "I have to admit that I always thought I had a difficult child," said one father. "After the tubes were put in, he became a delightful child. I began to like him a lot better."

TAKING SPECIAL CARE OF EARS
WITH TUBES ━━━━━━━━━━━━━━━━━━

Getting Water in the Ears

Most doctors recommend special care be taken to prevent water from entering the ear canal because of the possibility of infection from bacteria carried through the tube to the middle ear. Other doctors disagree, and four recent studies question whether protection is needed while swimming or bathing and have shown that many children do not get ear infections when they do not wear ear plugs. [1,2,3]

No consensus has been reached among ear specialists about whether children should wear tubes while swimming or bathing. If your child does not object to using ear canal protectors then it might be wise to avoid water in the ears to prevent possible infection.

Other Precautions

Call your doctor if your child develops pain in his ears, has excessive drainage from the ear, or has difficulty hearing or bleeds from the ears (this happens if an extruding tube causes granulation tissue or abrasion of skin in the ear canal). Some doctors may instruct you to put drops in the child's ears for a few days after surgery to prevent dried blood from clotting the hollow opening of the tube. Otherwise, no special precautions are needed.

Follow-Up Care for the Child With Tubes

A tympanostomy tube is a foreign substance implanted in the body. Although the tubes are made of materials which have been tested and found to cause minimal or no adverse body reaction, they cannot be neglected or forgotten. Therefore, a child with tympanostomy tubes should have an ear examination at least every six months until the tubes have become extruded or are surgically removed, the eardrum has healed, and a hearing test demonstrates normal hearing. Usually, this is done by the ear doctor who inserted the tubes, though follow-up care can be provided by the primary care physician.

The doctor will check the position of the tube, whether it is open, and the condition of the eardrum. Sometimes, the tube can irritate adjacent portions of the eardrum, which leads to the formation of a "foreign body reaction" and development of a red inflammatory growth of body tissue called "granulation tissue."

If your child had hearing impairment before the tubes were inserted, then she probably will have a follow-up hearing test during the first post-operative visit.

Extrusion of the Tube

As the eardrum replenishes its surface layer, the tube in the ear gradually works its way out of the eardrum. Generally, it is best for the tube to come out by itself gradually so the eardrum can slowly heal around the tube as it emerges. The doctor will not remove a tube that is still partially in the eardrum because removal would be painful and might tear the eardrum.

Reinserting the Tubes

Tympanostomy tubes do not "cure" a child's chronic condition; rather, they provide an artificial means of ventilation for the middle ear while the child's body continues to grow and mature. After the tube has fallen out of the eardrum, the child's middle ear problems can recur, and, in some cases, tubes may have to be reinserted.

However, the great majority of children do not need reinsertion of the tubes because by the time the tubes have come out, the child's eustachian tube should be functioning better than when the tubes were inserted. Put simply, the child will likely have outgrown a need for tubes.

Unless a tube has come out of a child's ear within a few weeks after insertion, the ear doctor will usually wait several months before even considering reinsertion of tubes. If the child has outgrown the frequent ear infections, and does have recurrent accumulation of fluid in her ears, then she will not require reinsertion of tubes.

Even when a child does start having frequent ear infections, persistent fluid, or both, after a first set of tubes have come out, then, most likely, your pediatrician and ear specialist will try medication and wait a considerable length of time before even considering tubes for a second time. The doctors will look for reasons why the child hasn't outgrown the frequent infections. They might test her for allergies, and may try antibiotic medication. If medication does not help, and the doctors are recommending reinsertion of tubes, then you should compare your child's ear problems since the time that the tubes came out with the problems she had before the tubes were inserted. If the problems have diminished, then you might want to wait, because your child's condition just might be slowly improving as she gets older.

Concerns about multiple insertions of tubes weakening and scarring the eardrum are realistic. However, remember that multiple ear infections and longstanding persistent middle ear fluid can also cause structural damage to the middle ear ossicles and to the eardrum.

QUESTIONS AND ANSWERS

Q: After having tubes inserted, I noticed my child seemed to be frightened by high levels of noise, such as the vacuum cleaner. What causes this sensitivity to certain tones?

A: Your child probably now has an increased acuity for hearing. Also, the tube may interfere with a reflex that tenses the intact eardrum to protect the middle ear from loud noise.

Q: My doctor told me the tube was starting to come out of the eardrum. How can he tell this? Can he tell how long it will take before the tube actually comes out? Why doesn't he just take it out right away?

A: The doctor observes the position of the tube relative to the surface of the eardrum. As the tube begins to extrude, more of the tube becomes visible to the doctor. When almost all of the tube is visible, this means that the tube is almost entirely out of the eardrum. It is best for the tube to come out of the eardrum gradually so that the eardrum can slowly heal around the tube.

Q: If a tube has come out of the eardrum spontaneously and is in the ear canal, will it interfere with hearing or cause any other damage?

A: It will not interfere with hearing but it can cause itching and an uncomfortable sensation.

Q: What kind of ear plugs should my child use when she swims?

A: Several kinds that have been shown to be effective are: Mack's® ear plugs; "Doc's"® plugs; and custom-made molds (which are expensive).

Q: My friend's daughter had ear tubes inserted over a year ago and has had no problems whatsoever. But my son's ear tubes have continually been plugged by mucus. Why is it that some children's ear tubes get plugged while others don't?

A: There has been no scientific study to provide a satisfactory answer to this question. Possibly your son's mucus is thicker and contains more sugars produced by the body, thereby making the mucus stickier and more likely to cause plugging of the tympanostomy tube.

Q: What do I do if my child gets an ear infection while he has tubes in his ears?

A: If your child has an upper respiratory infection (common cold) and then you begin to see drainage from one or both ears, it is likely that the "ear infection" is caused by viral infection and thus should subside within a few days without requiring treatment with an antibiotic. Some doctors may recommend that you instill in your child's ear an antibiotic solution (suspension) that will reduce chances for bacterial growth in the ear and help prevent tenacious mucus from blocking the lumen of the tube.

NOTES

1.   Jaffe BF. Are Water and Tympanostomy Tubes Compatible? The Laryngoscope. 1981:91, 563–64.
2.   Marks NJ, Mills RP. Swimming and grommets. Journal of the Royal Society of Medicine. 1983 Jan:76, 23–26.
3.   Smelt GC, Yeoh LH. Swimming and grommets. Journal Laryng Otol. 1984 March:98, 243–245.

CHAPTER THREE

Discussion and Controversies About Ear Tubes

Impact on U.S. Society

Myringotomy with insertion of tympanostomy tubes is the most common minor surgical procedure performed on children in the United States. At least one million children annually have tubes inserted in their ears,[1] but the actual number is probably greater since outpatient surgical centers and hospitals that do outpatient surgery do not report the number and types of surgery.

Consequently, there is no reliable information as to how much money is being spent per year on surgery. It costs roughly $1,300 for the insertion of tubes in both ears in the operating room of a hospital or outpatient surgical center, but only $150 for insertion of two tubes in the doctor's office with local anesthesia. If three-fourths of the children undergo the procedure in the operating room, the cost would be $975 million, with an additional $37.5 million spent for procedures done in doctor's offices. Total annual cost could well be more than $1 billion.[2]

Do Tubes "Work"?
A Look at Studies on the Usefulness of Tubes

Many researchers have attempted to study the usefulness of tubes but no consensus has been reached regarding their effectiveness. This section includes an international sampling of recent studies on tubes that demonstrate the disparate results and opinions. Doctors put more credence in some studies than in others. Generally, the more objective the study and the greater the number of patients studied, the more reliable and helpful is the information.

Some studies on tubes are thorough and comprehensive while others report on very small groups of patients and draw conclusions difficult to interpret. Another problem occurs when a study reports on a seemingly-related, but actually irrelevant, topic. For example, a team may cite damage to the eardrums caused by tubes, implying that tubes may scar eardrums. Though this may occur, the impact of these scars on the eardrum is really what needs to be considered, rather than just their existence. If a child needed surgery to improve knee function, doctors would not consider surgery unworthwhile because the child would have a scar on the knee.

Another variable of studies about tubes is the question of how children's hearing is assessed. Some studies imply that tympanostomy tubes are not worthwhile because comparisons show that a group of children who had tubes inserted had hearing equal to that of a group who did not. However, those studies often report hearing was tested at the beginning of the study, and not after the tubes had come out. Often, the studies do not test the hearing at periodic intervals throughout the entire study period.

Study #1:

In a recently published report, Gunnar Stickler, M.D., of the Mayo Clinic, expresses skepticism about the use of tympanostomy tubes. He suggests that surgeons are seeking to benefit financially from the plethora of tube insertions and points out that most adults who had ear infections as children were not harmed by the treatment they received, which probably did not include tubes. In the summary of his report, Dr. Stickler states:

> *Could it be that 1 million children each year have un-necessary surgical procedures involving the tympanic membrane? Has the availability of third-party payments fostered the spreading use of these procedures? Is this another reason for the rising cost of medical care?*
>
> *Anyway, for a child with secretory otitis, the best help at this time seems to be a prescription called "tincture of time," fortified by the realization that many of us in practice today had fluid in our ears when we were children. Did it really cause a degree of retardation? If not, let us declare a moratorium on tube placements until solid data supporting the procedure have been reported.*[3]

Study #2:

In a report from England, Nick Black, M.D., points out an "epidemic" of surgery for glue ear (persistent middle ear fluid). He notes the increase in the number of operations for otitis media far exceeds any increase in the numbers of children being afflicted with persistent middle ear fluid. In suggesting that some of the operations (for insertion of tubes) might be unnecessary, Dr. Black writes:

> *Firstly, the magnitude of the changes in surgical rate in some health regions—74 percent in Oxford, 122 percent in E. Anglia—are unlikely to be a reflection solely of similar increases in disease prevalence. Chronic diseases do not undergo such dramatic fluctuations. Secondly, the highest rates of surgery were in upper social classes . . . the current epidemic of surgery for glue ear seems to reflect an apparent rather than real increase in the prev-*

alence of the condition being treated, and the rate of surgery continues to rise.[4]

Study #3:

This study involved placement of a tube (grommet type) in one ear of 54 children for treatment of persistent otitis media. Then, at different time intervals, results in the ear with a tube were compared to results in the ear without a tube. Results of the study are a bit difficult to interpret because all children underwent adenoidectomy at the same time that the tube was inserted.

The investigators reported:

Both sides improved and remained significantly improved at 12 months. At 3 months, the side with the grommet improved significantly more than the other side, but at 12 months there was no significant difference between the two sides.[5]

Study #4:

A similar study involving insertion of a tube in only one ear and comparison of results in both ears suggested that tympanostomy tubes must be used with great caution. The author of the report summarized the findings as follows:

It is concluded that the use of ventilation tubes in children with primary secretory otitis media is not justified. Observation has shown that only a small proportion will require surgical treatment of the middle ear. A ventilation tube may be indicated in order to combat hearing loss, but it should be borne in mind that its use involves a high risk of complications and sequelae which may result in chronic middle ear disease.[6]

Study #5:

A report from San Juan, Puerto Rico, said:

Ventilation tubes are of extreme value in the treatment of serous otitis media and in the prevention of dreadful complications to the ear and hearing mechanism. However, irresponsible use of ventilation tubes with improper follow-up (until the tubes have been removed or extruded) must be condemned. Complications arising from ventilation tubes should be promptly corrected to avoid permanent damage to an otherwise healthy patient.[7]

Study #6:

A report funded by the well respected House Ear Institute in Los Angeles summarized findings as follows:

We reviewed the indications for and complications of myringotomy and ventilation tube placement in 1,099 patients over a 6-year period. There were 2,266 intubations and reintubations.

The most common indications were otitis media with effusion and recurrent acute otitis media. In 7 percent the indication was not related to otitis media.

Brief episodes of otorrhea (discharge) occurred in 19 percent and were much less common in those 7 percent who did not have underlying otitis media. Profuse persistent discharge occurred in 2 percent. Two patients required mastoid surgery for control of the infection.[8]

Study #7:

A study from Israel shows tubes helpful in management for children who seem unable to outgrow ear infections because of abnormal eustachian tube function:

Long-term V.T. (ventilation tube) in ears with non-curable eustachian dysfunction may be kept in place permanently as a treatment of choice. This treatment may assist in preparing some of the ears for elective surgery if and when indicated. It may also help overcome the tendency of the disease to recur following reconstructive middle ear and mastoid surgery.

It is not contended that long-term ventilation is curative in nature or that it always reverses the disease process, but rather that it helps to check the disease before it reaches the point of no return.[9]

Study #8:

Dr. Gordon D.L. Smyth, a world renowned ear surgeon from Ireland, recently reviewed the treatment of otitis media with effusion. He reported that the type of tube used greatly affected success:

The point must be made that the reported results of tympanostomy, when it is correctly performed and adequately monitored, surpass all other therapies for OME (otitis media with effusion) because it will immediately, in three-quarters of ears, and eventually in practically all ears, prevent the very real and serious consequences of enzymatic damage to the tympanic membrane (eardrum) and ossicular chain.[10]

Study #9:

In a study done in Italy, it appears that tympanostomy tubes are beneficial as long as the patients are well selected. The Italian investigators also suggest that adenoidectomy is helpful:

(1) The results appear to justify the methodology (insertion of tubes) and the inconveniences do not go against this, provided (a) insertion of the tympanostomy tube is

performed only in otitis-prone children . . . where adequate medical therapy failed to give lasting results, (b) the surgical technique employed is correct.

(2) Whenever indicated, adenoidectomy is performed at the same time, as it appears to improve the positive effects.[11]

Study #10:

A survey of a large number of ear specialists suggests that tympanostomy tubes do reduce the frequency of ear infections and benefits of the tubes outweigh risks; still there are some skeptics:

Experience with ventilating tubes extending over a period of 30 years has been compared twice with computer-assisted analysis of questionnaires submitted to 500 prominent, well-qualified otolaryngologists practicing throughout the world. Tubes were used by 99.4 percent of the respondents in 1982, and the consensus is that appropriate use of tubes has brought about a reduction in the incidence of chronic ear disease. Benefits from tympanostomy tubes far outweigh the very small number of tube-induced complications . . . from a few dissenting voices, and they are few indeed, we have heard that ventilating tubes are without value and may even do more harm than good. The vast majority of us disagree.[12]

Study #11:

One major ongoing study at the Children's Hospital of Pittsburgh is attempting to evaluate the effectiveness of tubes. Early results show that insertion of tubes gave the child less time with ear disease and hearing loss during a one-year period than did either myringotomy without tube insertion or no surgery.[2]

Study #12:

George Gates, M.D., head of the Division of Otolaryngology at the University of Texas Health Science Center, along with coinvestigators, recently completed a study on the effectiveness of tympanostomy and summarized the results of the well designed and comprehensive study as follows:

> *To investigate the therapeutic efficacy of current treatments of . . . otitis media, the authors undertook a randomized clinical trial with four treatment arms: myringotomy alone, tympanostomy tubes, adenoidectomy and myringotomy, and the combination of adenoidectomy and tympanostomy tubes. This report describes the preliminary (one-year) outcome in the group of children who were treated with tympanostomy tubes. The observed average differences between the myringotomy and tympanostomy tube groups were small . . . Although the clinical importance of these differences remains to be established, the authors believe they are substantial enough to justify continued use of tympanostomy tubes in the primary surgical therapy of . . . otitis media, when medical therapy and observation indicate the need for drainage to improve hearing or correct anatomic deformities of the eardrum.* [13]

Risks Versus Benefits: What Do the Experts Say?

The lack of consensus about the effectiveness of tubes has led Charles Bluestone, M.D., and Jerome Klein, M.D., to comment in *Pediatric Otolaryngology*: "No randomized clinical trial of the efficacy of myringotomy with tympanostomy tube insertion has been reported . . . it is important to know if the beneficial effects of tympanostomy tube insertion outweigh potential complications and sequelae." [14]

Because of the possible adverse effects, some experts are very cautious in recommending insertion of tubes. As Gordon Smyth, M.D., commented in the *American Journal of Otology*:

"every time a set of tubes is put in, the doctor is heightening risks of irreversible damage.[10] T. Lindholdt, M.D., in a Scandinavian journal, counsels against the use of tubes in children suffering middle ear fluid: "Use of tubes in children with otitis media is not justified. Its use involves a high risk of complication and sequalea which may result in chronic otitis media."[6]

Other experts argue against overreacting to the adverse effects of tubes. Jack L. Paradise, M.D., of the Children's Hospital of Pittsburgh, comments: "In most instances, the damage to the eardrum does not cause significant hearing loss; adverse effects may be due to the underlying disease rather than the tubes; and had tubes not been used, the diseased condition may have been worse."[1]

Another question that researchers are asking is: What, if any, are the long-term adverse effects of tubes? Will scarring or atrophy cause problems for children as they grow older? Since this generation's children are the first to undergo tube insertion in such large numbers, researchers have not completed followup studies to determine what long-term effects the treatment has on a child as he gets older.

Risks Versus Benefits: How's a Parent to Decide?

Most experts agree tubes "work" while they are in place by allowing for normal hearing and by possibly preventing structural damage to the middle ear that has a chronic condition.[15] Conversely, there is little evidence tubes prevent a chronic condition after they come out, and it is known that tubes can damage the eardrum and can cause excessive drainage or fail to work.

How does a parent weigh the benefits of tube insertion with the possible risks? Certainly, there are cases with a clearcut answer, such as the two-and-one-half-year-old child who can barely speak because of hearing loss as a result of middle ear fluid.

But many, many cases are not clear cut. The parent and physician will need to discuss thoroughly the risks and benefits of tympanostomy tubes as they pertain to the individual child. As discussed previously, this is not an urgent decision and should be made only after careful monitoring of the child's condition and if a course of preventive antimicrobial treatment has failed to clear up persistent middle ear fluid or reduce the frequency of episodes of otitis media.

Although they say that ". . . clinical trials are urgently needed to confirm this apparent success (of insertion of tympanostomy tubes),"[14] Charles Bluestone, M.D., and Jerome Klein, M.D., in the textbook *Pediatric Otolaryngology*, continue:

> *"It does not seem the use of tympanostomy tubes is a modern fad that will become obsolete in the near future . . . since insertion of tympanostomy tubes permits hearing preservation and probably prevents many of the complications and sequelae of otitis media while the tubes are in place, their use is advocated despite the fact that otitis media usually improves with increasing age."*[15]

QUESTIONS AND ANSWERS

Q: Is it true insertion of tympanostomy tubes is rapidly replacing tonsillectomy and adenoidectomy as the most popular operation for children? If so, why?

A: Insertion of tympanostomy tubes has become the most commonly performed minor surgical procedure in children while the frequency with which tonsillectomy and adenoidectomy are performed has rapidly declined. The reasons are as follows: (1) The use of antibiotics in the treatment of tonsillitis and ear infections means there is less need to remove children's tonsils to cure frequent strep sore throats; (2) In the past 10 years, doctors have developed stringent indications for tonsillectomy and adenoidectomy (T&A) resulting in fewer T&A operations being performed; (3) New technology enables greater ease in insertion of tympanostomy tubes, such as the use of the operating microscope for ear surgery and mass production of individually wrapped sterile non-reactive tympanostomy tubes; (4) Mass screening of children's hearing, widespread use of sophisticated, but easy to use audiometric test equipment and common use of diagnostic equipment to detect otitis media has resulted in more children being diagnosed as having ear infection.

Q: My pediatrician is quite emphatic in his opinion that tympanostomy tubes are not good for children. He refers less than 10 children each year to have tubes put in their ears, and says there are numerous reports in prestigious medical journals clearly stating children do not greatly benefit from insertion of tubes and the risks with tubes outweigh the benefits. Is all this true?

A: There have been numerous reports in medical journals suggesting that tympanostomy tubes are not very effective or helpful in management of children's ear infections. However, by no means are all the reports negative. Several well-designed scientific studies have shown that tympanostomy tubes can be quite helpful for many children. This chapter includes a sampling of the most recent reports in medical journals regarding the usefulness of inserting tympanostomy tubes in children's ears. From reading the excerpts, you will see that the matter of inserting tympanostomy tubes is controversial. Pediatricians and family physicians should not take a single-minded approach to the issue of ear infections; every child should be evaluated individually and may, or may not, benefit from the insertion of ear tubes.

Q: My son Jason has had frequent ear infections for the past two years and his hearing usually isn't good because of the almost constant fluid in his ears. Several times I have asked the pediatrician to refer him for evaluation by an ENT specialist, but the pediatrician keeps saying that Jason doesn't need to see the specialist and insists he doesn't need tubes in his ears. I think the pediatrician is reluctant to refer Jason and he considers my repeated requests an affront. What should I do?

A: *Discuss your concerns with your pediatrician and your reasons for wanting the opinion of an ENT specialist. It is doubtful he actually would be offended, especially once he is fully aware of your concerns and frustrations. Make a list of your concerns and ask your pediatrician to spend sufficient time with you to answer your questions. Also, remember that an ENT specialist should not be viewed merely as an "installer of tubes"; he is a doctor trained specifically in management of ear disorders and may be able to offer several alternatives which can help in managing your child's ear infections.*

NOTES

1. Paradise JL. On Tympanostomy Tubes: Rationale, Results, Reservations and Recommendations. Pediatrics. 1977 July: 60 (1): 86–90.

2. Mandel EM, Bluestone CD, Paradise JL, Cantekin EI, et al. "Efficacy of Myringotomy With and Without Tympanostomy Tube Insertion in the Treatment of Chronic Otitis Media with Effusion in Infants and Children: Results for the First Year of a Randomized Clinical Trial" in Recent Advances in Otitis Media With Effusion (DJ Lim, editor-in-chief). B.C. Decker, 1984: 308–312.

3. Stickler GB. The Attack on the Tympanic Membrane. Pediatrics. 1984 Aug: 74(2); 291–292.

4. Black N. Surgery for Glue Ear—A Modern Epidemic. The Lancet. 1984 Apr 14:835–37.

5. To SS, Pahor AL, Robin PE. A prospective trial of unilateral grommets for bilateral secretory otitis media in children. Clin Otolaryngol. 1984 Apr; 9(2):115–17.

6. Lindholdt T. Ventilation Tubes in Secretory Otitis Media. A randomized, controlled study of the course, complications and sequaelae of ventilation tubes. Acta Otol (Suppl) Stock 1983: 398: 1–28.

7. Fernandez-Blasini N. Use and Abuse of Ventilation Tubes. American Journal of Otology. 1985 March: 6(2), 142–43.

8. Luxford WM, Sheehy JL. Ventilation Tubes: Indications and Complications. American Journal of Otology. 1984 Oct:5(6), 468–471.

9. Eliachar I, Joachims HZ, Goldsher M, Golz A. Assessment of Long-term Middle Ear Ventilation. Acta Otolaryngol 1983: 96,105–112.

10. Smyth G. Management of Otitis Media With Effusion: A Review. The American Journal of Otology. 1984 July; 5(5): 344–349.

11. Fior R, Veljak C. Late results and complications of tympanostomy tube insertion for prophylaxis of recurrent purulent otitis media in pediatric age. International J of Pediatric Otorhinolaryngology. 8(1984) 139–146.

12. Armstrong BW, Armstrong RB. Ventilating Tubes Are the Treatment of Choice for Nonsupparative Otitis Media. Amer J Otol. 1984 Jan: 5(3), 250–252.

13. Gates GA, Wachtendorf C, Hearne EM, Holt GR. Treatment of Chronic Otitis Media with Effusion: Results of Tympanostomy Tubes. American J Otolaryngology. 1985 May:6(3):249–253.

14. Bluestone CD, Klein JO. "Otitis Media with Effusion, Atelectasis and Eustachian Tube Dysfunction" in Pediatric Otolaryngology Volume 1 (edited by CD Bluestone and SE Stool). 1983 WB Saunders Co.: 480.

(15) Bluestone CD, Klein JO. "Otitis Media with Effusion, Atelectasis and Eustachian Tube Dysfunction" in Pediatric Otolaryngology Volume 1 (edited by CD Bluestone and SE Stool). 1983 WB Saunders Co.: 486.

PART SIX

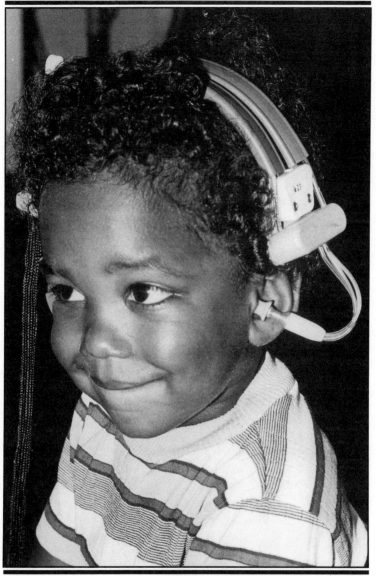

Hearing Loss

CHAPTER ONE

The Connection Between Ear Infections and Hearing Loss

For several months before birth, the fetus hears the sounds around him: the swoosh of the amniotic fluid, the beat of his mother's heart, and perhaps even voices and music emanating from outside the womb. However, at the moment of birth, the child is immediately bombarded with countless unfamiliar sounds, and perhaps comforted by the familiar sounds of his mother's voice and the beat of her heart as she embraces him. The newborn is like a sponge who indiscriminately absorbs all the sounds in his environment. Within a few days of birth, the infant begins to attach meaning to the sounds of feeding, the sounds of comfort, the sounds of distress. During the first years of life, hearing enables the child to associate meaning with words, sounds with the objects that make them, and voices with people. Without hearing, the child is at a distinct disadvantage in making sense of the complex world around him.

Intermittent hearing loss is common in children with persistent middle ear fluid and the American Academy of Pediatrics says "it is important that the physician inform the parent that a child with middle ear disease may not hear normally." The duration of this hearing loss can be from one day to several months; can be slight or moderate; and may or may not be detected by parents. In some cases, intermittent hearing loss can result in delayed speech and language as well as social and academic problems.

Today, the question of whether hearing loss from middle ear fluid results in developmental delays is a controversial one debated among pediatricians, otolaryngologists, audiologists, speech-language pathologists and educators. Despite numerous studies, little consensus has been reached on how the individual child is affected by fluctuating hearing loss.

The lack of agreement in this area is one reason why there is such a wide range of treatment for children who suffer persistent middle ear fluid. Physicians who believe that intermittent hearing loss results in speech and language delay will be more rigorous in their treatment; these specialists may be over-referring children for hearing, medical and speech-language evaluation. At the other extreme are physicians who are seemingly unconcerned about the hearing loss that can accompany chronic otitis media; these physicians may delay many months before referring children for evaluation—or they may never make a referral.

If your child is suffering intermittent hearing loss as a result of persistent middle ear fluid, should you be concerned that her language, speech and educational development might be delayed? There is little need to worry if your child suffers an occasional ear infection. Only if your child suffers persistent middle ear fluid would it be wise for you to monitor your child's hearing. But you should not assume that your child will suffer developmental delays from persistent middle ear fluid. The consequences of hearing loss are different for each child; two children who have middle ear fluid for three months will react differently.

Medical decisions, therefore, cannot be generalized, because the consequences of middle ear fluid on hearing are different for every child. An important guideline to use regarding medical decisions is to establish a baseline evaluation of the child's hearing and/or speech and language if the child suffers chronic ear problems. For example, if your child has middle ear fluid for more than three months, a hearing test will help determine whether any loss has occurred and how much. That test will be compared with future hearing tests as the child's illness is monitored.

Two examples illustrate the different ways otitis media can affect hearing:

After four ear infections in three months, 2-year-old Matthew was referred to an ENT specialist, who detected fluid in both ears. A hearing test showed a 20 dB hearing loss in each ear and a tympanogram indicated the presence of fluid. The parents detected no problem in Matthew's speech development and said Matthew complained of no discomfort as a result of the fluid. Therefore, the ENT specialist decided to wait six weeks, at which time he would reexamine the ears and request another hearing test. On that follow-up visit, the ENT specialist found fluid in only one ear and observed that the other eardrum had returned to normal. At that point, the specialist said he was not overly concerned about Matthew's hearing because it was probably good at least in one ear. Finally, after an additional four weeks, the ear which had persistent fluid returned to a normal appearance and a second hearing test was normal for both ears.

Carolyn is a 4-year-old who was referred to an ENT specialist after a hearing loss was detected in a preschool screening test. The specialist found fluid in both ears, and a hearing test showed 25 dB hearing loss in both ears. The parents agreed Carolyn's speech was not as advanced as her peers' and that they often thought Carolyn was not hearing well, but attributed it to deliberate inattentiveness by Carolyn. The ENT specialist anesthesized and then lanced Carolyn's eardrums to release the fluid, prescribed prophylactic antibiotics to help prevent the fluid from returning, and advised the parents that Carolyn might have to have tubes inserted in her ears if the fluid recurred withing three months. Carolyn also was referred to a speech-language therapist for evaluation and possible therapy.

As illustrated in the above examples, medical decisions should be approached carefully and should take into account the findings of a medical examination, the results of hearing tests, and speech and language skills.

Effects of Hearing Loss

The soft sounds your child hears when he has middle ear fluid means he may be able to understand some of what you're saying, but he can't distinguish the subtle sounds of speech that contribute to the meaning of language. Inflections and short words spoken rapidly may not be heard.

Once the fluid clears from their ears, most children will be able to compensate for these missed opportunities and catch up to peers without any permanent delay. However, other children may miss out on an important link in the chain of language development. These children may begin to experience trouble once they're in a classroom and have to decipher increasingly complex types of verbal communication.

How much of a hearing loss must occur before a problem develops? The answer is unknown. Factors such as the child's environment and intelligence play a role in how he will be affected by hearing loss. However, some researchers have attempted to determine the approximate decibel level at which understanding of speech becomes confused. They claim that children with a hearing loss of 40 decibels or less apparently have no difficulty adjusting in the classroom—they simply

---

Effects of Intermittent Hearing Loss

- Socialization
- Parent/child relationship
- Speech/language development
- Learning problems

cannot process "faint" speech. However, these researchers estimate that articulation problems and speech discrimination problems may occur with a hearing loss from 41–55 dB.[2] Others say losses between 25 dB and 40 dB after the first year of life may interfere with articulation.[1]

Researchers suspect a child could be affected by intermittent hearing loss as a result of persistent middle ear fluid in the following areas:

Socialization/Education. A child who is falling behind his peers in speech skills and who cannot hear everything in his classroom may begin to experience problems in academic or social areas of his life. Since the child who is suffering ear discomfort and hearing loss may become distracted and mischievous in a classroom, behavioral problems may develop.

Parent-Child Relationship. The younger child may have no other way to express his discomfort than by lashing out at other children, acting irritably, or seeking attention through misbehavior. This irritability, whining, uncooperativeness or other disagreeable behavior may lead parents to consider their child "difficult" and could affect the parent/child relationship.

One mother who didn't realize her daughter was suffering a hearing loss said, "We thought we were letting her get away with too many things because she was sick so often." The mother explained that Heather was having problems at school, fighting with other children and coming home and telling her parents that she was a "bad girl." The mother continued,

So we really tried cracking down. There were a couple of weeks there when we were really mean to her. But when Heather was examined by an ENT specialist, fluid was found in both ears and a hearing test showed moderate loss of hearing in the right ear and slight loss of hearing in the left ear. I feel so guilty now, not realizing the discomfort she felt and the hearing loss she was experiencing.

Speech development. Effects of temporary hearing loss are subtle. For example, when listening to a parent speak, the child may not distinguish between the words "places" or "placed." Many children will be able to discern these differences once the fluid clears. But for the child who may not learn some of these distinctions, the problems can be ultimately reflected in delayed speech and/or reading skills.

Language and learning problems. Some 30 studies involving 3,500 children have shown a consistent association of early fluctuating hearing losses with later decreased learning skills. In and of itself, each study was inconclusive, and most professionals find some fault with each study.[3] The very presence of the plethora of studies in this area, however, suggest that the question is a valid one that needs to be answered. (See discussion of research below.)

Hearing loss caused by structural damage to the middle ear. See page 87 for discussion of adverse effects of otitis media.

Children Most at Risk for Developing Problems From Hearing Loss

A major challenge facing specialists who care for children with hearing loss is determining which children will suffer educational and social delays as a result of fluctuating hearing loss. Many factors play a role in how a child will adjust to hearing loss, and many of these factors cannot be measured by a simple test.

Some of these include:

- Do the child's parents reinforce and encourage speech?
- Is there stress at home that may interfere with normal development?
- Does the child miss a great deal of social activity (such as play groups or preschool) because of illness?
- Is the child receiving proper medical care?

The child with normal to superior intelligence may develop good listening skills that will help him compensate for intermittent hearing loss. If this child is in a home where communication is encouraged and stimulated, where the parental bond is strong and where the child is exposed to many different places and people, then she probably will not suffer delay because of mild hearing loss. However, an unanswered and possibly unanswerable question remains: Is the child's potential achievement diminished by intermittent hearing loss from persistent middle ear fluid?

The child at a most distinct disadvantage is the child with low to normal intelligence who may be in a family in which he is not receiving abundant language and learning experiences or good medical care. Another child at a disadvantage is the child who suffers multiple physical or emotional handicaps in addition to chronic otitis media.

RESEARCH ON OTITIS MEDIA AND HEARING LOSS

Researchers are asking the questions: How much hearing loss, and for how long, is tolerable in the young child? Does hearing loss affect children differently at different ages? Are there permanent effects from temporary hearing loss? What role does the child's family life play in the impact of hearing loss? Is hearing loss in one ear relatively innocuous? Or could it be harmful?

Experts welcomed a study published in August 1984 in *Pediatrics*, citing its results and claiming that the study's design met the strict standards of scientific method.[4] Reported by D.W. Teele, M.D., J.O. Klein, M.D., et al., the study says that children who spent prolonged periods of time with middle ear fluid scored lower on tests of speech and language at age three than did children who spent little or no time with middle ear fluid. The researchers also showed that time spent with middle ear fluid in the first year of life was most strongly associated with lower scores on tests of speech and language.

But even the researchers had unanswered questions. They said they did not know if the poor test scores would persist through later years of life, nor if these children would recover and perform as well as children who did not have persistent middle ear fluid. The researchers also were unable to determine if parent-child stimulation, or the effect of chronic illness on this stimulation, could have accounted for some of the observed differences between the two groups of children.

Since the publication of the Teele-Klein study, one study in the *New England Journal of Medicine* reported that although persistent middle ear fluid may result in hearing and speech impairment, the data do not support the hypothesis that cognitive, language and psychosocial development are adversely affected.[5] Yet another study since published in *Pediatrics* in January 1986 by Jack Paradise, M.D., and Kenneth Rogers, M.D., says the Teele-Klein study's "findings appear largely not to support the authors' intepretations, inferences and conclusions."[6]

Another recent study says that infants with recurrent otitis media may be considered at high risk for developmental language disorders. A group of infants who had suffered ear infections scored lower in tests for acquiring speech skills as compared with a group of infants who did not have such frequent otitis media. The authors suggest that these infants may need early language stimulation to offset possible language problems.

NOTES ═══════════════════════════════════════

1. Northern JL, Lemme J: Hearing and auditory disorders, in Shames G, Wiig E (eds): *Human Communications Disorders*. Columbus, OH, Charles E Merrill Publishing Co., 1982: 299–329.

2. Menyuk P. Design Factors in the Assessment of Language Development in Children with Otitis media. Annals of Otol, Rhin, Laryng. 1979 Sept–Oct; Suppl 60:88(5–2):78–87.

3. Downs M. "Audiologist's Overview of Sequelae of Early Otitis Media" in Workshop on Effects of Otitis Media on Children. Pediatrics. 1983 April:71(4):643.

4. Teele DW, Klein JO, Rosner BH, et al. Otitis Media with Effusion During the First Three Years of Life and Development of Speech and Language. Pediatrics. 1984 Aug:74 (2).

5. Hubbard TW, Paradise JL, McWilliams BJ, et al. Consequences of Unremitting Middle Ear Disease in Early Life. The New England Journal of Medicine. 1985 June 13:312(24):1529–1534.

6. Paradise JL, Rogers KD. On Otitis Media, Child Development and Tympanostomy Tubes: New Answers or Old Questions? Pediatrics. 1986 Jan:77(1):88–92.

7. Ina F. Wallace, Ph.D.; Gravel, J.S.; McCarton, C.M.; Ruben, R.J. Otitis Media, Auditory Sensitivity and Language Outcomes at One Year. Laryngoscope. 1988 Jan:98(1):64-70 and Otitis Media and Language Development at One Year of Age. Journal of Speech and Hearing Disorders. 1988 Aug:53:245-251.

CHAPTER TWO

How We Hear

The ear is a sophisticated instrument, finely tuned and brilliantly engineered. We "hear" as a result of a series of physical, mechanical and electrical functions. It's a phenomenon we often take for granted until a link in the hearing chain is broken.

Sound is a form of energy produced when a movement causes a chain reaction of molecules bumping against one another. When you snap your fingers, the ensuing force presses against the molecules of air surrounding your fingertips. These molecules bump against their neighbors, and then return to their original space.

The action generated by all this "bumping" travels at about 1,000 feet per second and is called a sound wave. The faster each air molecule receives and causes a bump, the greater the frequency of sound. A high-pitched sound has a greater frequency than a low-pitched sound. Frequency is measured in cycles, or number of vibrations, per second (Cps) or Hertz (Hz). The harder you snap your fingers, the greater the intensity of the sound; the greater the intensity, the louder the sound. Intensity is measured in ratios and is the basis of the decibel (dB) scale.

Our ears are sensitive to only certain ranges of frequency and intensity: from 20 Hz (lower than the lowest notes of a

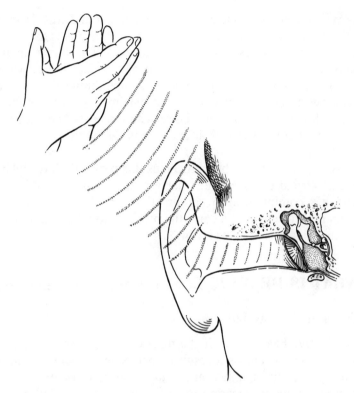

The transmission of sound waves is depicted with the clapping of hands. As the molecules vibrate against one another, they send energy to the ear canal. That energy vibrates the eardrum, which sends vibrations through the ossicles into the inner ear.

bass fiddle) to 20,000 Hz (beyond the upper reaches of a flute). A sound 10 times more intense than another at the same frequency differs by 10 dB; a sound 100 times more intense differs by 20 dB. For example, a whisper is about 20 dB, and normal conversation about 60 dB. Remember, when your child has an ear infection, or when fluid is present in his ear, your child may be suffering a hearing loss ranging from 15 dB to 40 dB, which is considered a mild or moderate loss.[1]

When you call your child's name, the sound travels from your mouth to your child's outer ear, which channels the sound energy and focuses it onto the eardrum. The bones in the middle ear convert this energy into mechanical force, which presses against the oval window. A membrane in the oval window bulges into the inner ear, where the sound vibrates through the inner ear fluid. Those vibrations stir the "touch" cells, which send electrical energy via the auditory nerves to the brain.

When your child's brain receives this message, it deciphers the electrical code and tells her that the sound is your voice and it's coming from a certain direction. Nerves from this sound-interpreting area carry the message to other parts of her brain, so she can answer you.

WHAT IS HEARING LOSS? ════════

Types of Hearing Loss

Conductive hearing loss is the most common form of hearing loss that can occur as a result of persistent middle ear fluid. An obstruction or infection in either the outer or middle ear causes conductive hearing loss. For instance, wax filling the ear canal can cause conductive hearing loss; or, with otitis media and effusion, the fluid interferes with the vibration of the tiny ossicles and diminishes the ability of the eardrum to vibrate. Conductive hearing loss usually is reversible. When a child's persistent middle ear fluid clears, his hearing will almost always return to normal.

Other types of hearing loss are: (1) sensorineural, which occurs when the inner ear is damaged and is almost always irreversible; and (2) mixed hearing loss, a combination of conductive and sensorineural. Approximately one of 750 infants have significant sensorineural bilateral hearing loss in both ears at birth or soon thereafter, and another six out of 1,000 will be identified as having significant sensorineural loss in early childhood. Possible causes of congenital sensorineural hearing loss include inherited factors, low birth weight, prematurity, meningitis, asphyxia and severe jaundice.

Severity of Hearing Loss

Degree of hearing loss is measured in decibels (dB) and can be graded in severity as follows:

Mild hearing loss:	20 dB to30 dB
Moderate:	31 dB to 60 dB
Severe:	61 dB to 80 dB

Unilateral and Bilateral Hearing Loss

Sometimes, your child will have fluid behind only one eardrum. This can produce unilateral hearing loss—that is, a loss of hearing in one ear only. Most audiologists believe a child with unilateral hearing loss hears well enough to function without difficulty in most situations. He may have trouble localizing the direction of sounds, but this problem may surface only when he is in large noisy crowds or in the classroom.

What Does It Feel Like to Have Fluid in the Ear?

A child whose middle ear is filled with fluid may experience a ''stopped up'' sensation similar to the feeling an adult gets just before his ears ''pop'' when taking off or landing in a plane. If this sensation is accompanied by hearing loss, sound for this child is very soft or muffled and is similar to the sounds one hears when the ears are filled with water after bathing or swimming. If you place a finger in each ear, you can get an idea of what your child is most likely experiencing when he has fluid in his ears.

Surprisingly, children are usually unaware they are suffering a hearing loss; they are content with the soft sounds that make up their hearing world. They adjust quickly to the hearing loss and, therefore, parents may never know that a hearing loss exists, especially when it's a very mild loss. As one mother explained: "To my son, it's just the normal flow of things; he doesn't notice he's not hearing right."

NOTE

1.   Northern JL, Lemme J. "Hearing and Auditory Disorders" in Human Communication Disorders (G Shames and E. Wiig, editors). 1982: Charles E. Merrill Pub. Co.: 299–329.

CHAPTER THREE

Detection

THE PARENT: SUSPECTING HEARING LOSS

For many children, the very mild hearing loss that can result from fluid in the ear may never be detected. Parents and children alike compensate for the hearing loss—probably without even realizing they're doing it. For instance, the parent may speak louder, repeat sentences or words, or may move closer to the child. The child compensates by watching a speaker's lips, moving closer to the sound, or asking the speaker to repeat himself. One telltale sign of hearing loss is when a child turns up the volume on a television set or record player in order to hear better.

Often, parents don't know if the child is deliberately ignoring them, or if he truly has a hearing loss. "I tell other mothers that I'd call my child, and he wouldn't respond," explained one mother whose son was found to have a hearing loss during a school screening test. "And the mothers would say, Well, my child does that all the time. That's how all 3- and 4-year-olds behave.' "

However, the child who has persistent middle ear fluid should be watched closely by the parent, examined regularly by a physician and tested periodically for hearing loss. Parents should be alert to any changes in the child's speech or behavior that indicates the hearing loss is interfering with the way the child speaks, learns language or perceives the world.

A speech and language screening chart included at the end of this section will help you determine whether your child's language acquisition is proceeding normally. Additionally, the parent can follow his own instincts—and these few guidelines—to determine whether hearing loss is significant:

- Does the child often ask you to repeat?
- Does the child easily follow directions?
- Does he often seem to be ignoring you or inattentive?
- Does his teacher or caretaker report listening or attention problems in school or in a playgroup?
- Is his speech unclear to others?
- If your child is an infant, does he turn in the direction of a loud noise?
- Is he startled by a sudden noise?
- Is the infant comforted by soothing words from someone familiar to him?

The alert parent can circumvent speech delays by monitoring the child's language development with a health professional. The earlier the hearing loss is detected and addressed, the easier it is to reverse or avoid any developmental delays or educational problems.[1]

THE PEDIATRICIAN OR FAMILY PHYSICIAN: PRELIMINARY TESTS

If you suspect your child may suffer hearing loss severe enough to impair speech or learning, discuss your concerns with the child's doctor. A doctor may be able to determine if formal assessment of hearing and speech-language development is needed. Unfortunately, some physicians tend to ignore parental concerns about their children's hearing: in one study of 300 children who suffered severe deafness, the average age at which the mother suspected and reported a hearing loss was 11 months; but the average age at which the losses were diagnosed was almost two-and-one-half years.[2] Consequently, it's important for parents to act on their instincts. As one mother said, "It was my intuition my son wasn't hearing well. And I decided it was worth my time and effort to get it checked. My pediatrician kept saying to wait a few more months, but I felt he may be needlessly suffering hearing loss." This mother consulted an ENT specialist despite the pediatrician's reluctance to make a referral, and her son was shown to be suffering a speech/language delay due to hearing loss.

Detecting mild hearing loss without sophisticated equipment is difficult. However, your pediatrician may screen your child's hearing by producing a sound with a rattle, squeeze toy or bell held outside the child's peripheral vision. Tuning forks are effective only with an older child. A more sophisticated tool, the portable audiometers, may be used by some family physicians or pediatricians. Additionally, they may use the tympanometer to determine if the ear is full of fluid. Though this is not a hearing test, it may indicate a cause for possible hearing loss. (See more detailed discussion of tympanometry in section on Audiologist: Confirming Hearing Loss).

The Robert Wood Johnson Foundation funded programs at five universities around the country to train primary care physicians to recognize potential or existing communication disorders in their young patients.[3] The $3-million program was intended to train primary care physicians in recognizing warning signs of disability due to hearing, speech and language disorders. Many pediatricians were taught to recognize early language milestones; the use of the tympanometer; and proper noisemaker hearing screening. It is hoped that primary care physicians will eventually use these packages to better determine which children need more sophisticated tests.

Your child should be screened for possible hearing problems during well-baby visits even if you do not suspect hearing loss. In the first years of life, it is difficult for parents to detect mild or even moderate hearing loss because the child can respond to many everyday sounds, especially loud ones. If your child is suspected of hearing loss as a result of middle ear fluid, your physician can refer him to a speech-hearing center for hearing tests.

THE SCHOOL SCREENING

Most schools conduct screening programs for hearing and vision; in many cities throughout the United States, some test of hearing is required before kindergarten. Today, many preschool programs offer hearing tests for a fee for children as young as two years old. These preschool programs may use a local hearing center to test the children. If a child does not pass the screening test, the parents are urged to have the child examined by their physician and retested under controlled conditions (in soundproof rooms).

THE ENT SPECIALIST: MEDICAL DIAGNOSIS

Your doctor may refer your child to an otolaryngologist (an ear, nose and throat specialist) to determine the cause of the hearing loss. The specialist will examine your child's ears with a pneumatic otoscope or a microscope, and he will check the child's nose and mouth, as well as take a complete medical history of the child's ear, nose and throat problems. (For a complete discussion of examination, see page 64).

The specialist should be able to determine from his examination whether your child has fluid in her ear and if there is any medical condition that could be interfering with your child's hearing. His examination can be the first step in evaluating whether there is a hearing loss.

In most cases of chronic otitis media, the child has been referred to an ENT specialist for treatment of an ear disorder rather than detection of hearing loss. However, some children have persistent middle ear fluid without any bouts of acute otitis media or showing any signs of discomfort. One 4-year-old was found to be suffering moderate hearing loss after being tested in nursery school. The parent told the ENT specialist that she had noticed no signs of hearing loss, nor had the child complained of discomfort or pain. Upon examination, the specialist found both middle ears full of fluid. The specialist prescribed an antibiotic in low dosage for four weeks. But when the fluid persisted and was detected on a follow-up visit, the specialist recommended insertion of tubes. A repeat hearing test done two weeks after the tubes had been inserted showed normal hearing for both ears.

"It was a very hard decision for us to make," said the mother. "My son never complained of any ear discomfort and he never had ear infections. But I was afraid the loss of hearing would interfere with his speech and language development. I still have mixed feelings about the decision to put the tubes in and I don't think I will have them reinserted when they come out."

Some ENT specialists routinely refer children with persistent middle ear fluid for hearing tests. In this way, the specialist can monitor hearing loss over the period of chronic ear problems. It may be helpful to the physician in determining which treatment is working the best: for instance, does the child hear better after insertion of ventilation tubes? Or did his hearing improve after a month of prophylactic antibiotics?

THE AUDIOLOGIST: CONFIRMING HEARING LOSS

An audiologist is trained to evaluate the degree and type of hearing loss through behavioral and objective auditory tests, and through observation. The audiologist knows how to interpret the response of the child to each test, and understands what response is appropriate for each age. Also, she is able to observe the child's behavior and speech during normal conversation for clues about the child's hearing, speech-language and social development—all of which are factors in the child's hearing test.

An audiologist should have at least a master's degree in the field of audiology and should hold a Certificate of Clinical Competence from the American Speech and Hearing Association and/or a license to practice audiology in the state in which she works (if such a license is necessary). When seeking an audiologist, try to find someone who is trained specifically to work with children.

Children's hearing is evaluated using subjective and objective tests. The subjective (or behavioral) hearing tests include those in which the audiologist interprets the child's response to levels of tones or sounds. The objective tests most commonly performed on children are given with the use of a tympanometer. These tests, among other things, measure middle ear function. Another objective test, called brainstem evoked response audiometry, measures brainwave activity in response to sound.

Tests should take place in specially constructed soundproof rooms that eliminate outside noise. The audiologist may be in the same room as the child, or in an adjacent one, depending upon the test circumstances.

Testing the Child Under Age 3

The audiologist trained to work with children is an expert at "shaping" a child's behavior (called conditioned response) in

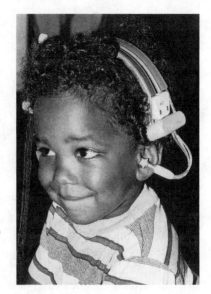

A child wearing the headpiece that is connected to the tympanometer. *(Photo by Cynthia J. Carney)*

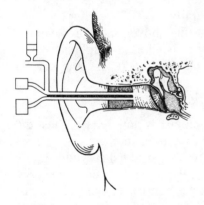

This illustration shows the position of the "acoustic bridge"— that part of the tympanometer which is placed in the ear canal to measure the function of the eardrum.

order to conduct subjective hearing tests. Before the audiologist starts conditioning for responses, however, she will chat with the parent and observe the child's behavior. She will listen to the child's voice quality and determine his articulation. All these factors play a part in assessment.

Subjective Testing. Here's one usual sequence of testing for children younger than 3: The first tests are conducted while the child and parent are in one soundproof room and the audiologist in an adjacent soundproof room. The two rooms are connected by a glass viewing panel so the audiologist can observe the child. The audiologist first conditions the child's behavior by pairing her voice (spoken through a microphone with speakers attached in the child's room) with the presence of an attractive toy that lights up in a corner of the room. When the child looks to that part of the room every time he hears the audiologist's voice, then the audiologist knows the child is conditioned. She then says words, or other vocalizations, like "ba ba" or "da da" at reducing levels of volume until the child no longer looks toward the toy. An audiometer is used to measure the sharpness and range of hearing through the use of controlled amounts of sound. Results of the test are recorded on a special type of graph called an audiogram.

For another test, the audiologist repeats the above sequence, except instead of speaking, she plays modulated pure tones over the speakers. She then repeats the entire process with earphones if the baby is cooperative.

A final test may repeat all of the above procedures using a bone oscillator. This instrument is like an earphone but is placed on the bone behind a child's ear. It tests the normal hearing of the inner ear and cochlea and can indicate potential middle ear problems or sensorineural hearing loss.

Objective Testing. The audiologist is now ready to test the function of the middle ear with a tympanometer. A special plug connected to earphones will be inserted in your child's ear. The plug sends tones down the ear canal, and the energy that is reflected back from the eardrum is measured by a calibrated microphone. One part of this testing that you may be familiar with is tympanometry. The eardrum's resistance to the tone is plotted by a curve on a piece of paper, called a tympanogram, as depicted in the illustrations on page 222. Ask the person who tests the child to show you the graph and explain the significance of the different curves.

Other tests that can be done through the use of the tym-

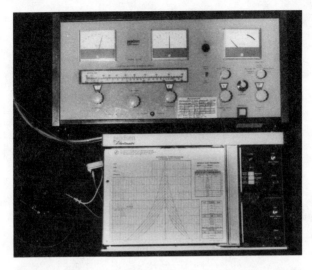

The tympanometer with its accompanying headpiece. The needle draws a curve on the chart that shows the function of the middle ear. *(Photo by Jerry A. McCoy)*

panometer are: (1) to measure the acoustic reflex (the reflex of the stapedial tendon that contracts to loud sounds); (2) to determine whether a tympanostomy tube is open or blocked; (3) to determine if the eustachian tube is functioning normally; and (4) to detect perforation in the eardrum.

To repeat: results of tympanometry tests are not a test of hearing, they are measurements of function of the middle ear and the eardrum. They should never be used as a sole means of diagnosing middle ear fluid. Rather, tympanometry results are used to confirm findings observed during careful examination of the eardrum.

Note: Though the tympanometer's plug is inserted only slightly into the child's ear canal, some children dislike any object being put into their ear. Test results obtained by a skilled audiologist, however, can be valid even if the baby is crying, moving or talking.

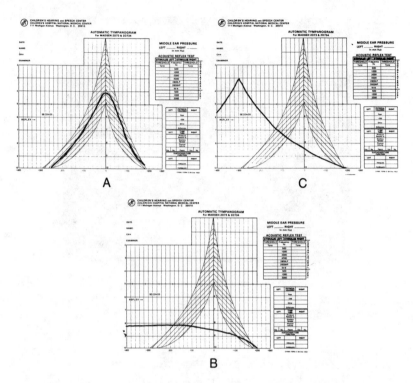

A

C

B

Above is shown the three classic curves of tympanogram patterns: Type A, B and C. Type A curves are found in patients with normal middle ear function; that is, air pressure is equal on both sides of the eardrum. Type B curves indicate that the eardrum is showing great resistance to sound and that fluid is most likely behind the ear. Type C curves show some mobility of the eardrum, and indicate that the eardrum is retracted, with or without the presence of fluid.

Testing the Child Between Age 3 and 5

The audiologist's tests for the preschooler are essentially the same, but she can now condition the child differently. Because the child is older, he will respond to "social" conditioning —that is, he will repeat an action if he is praised and en-

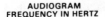

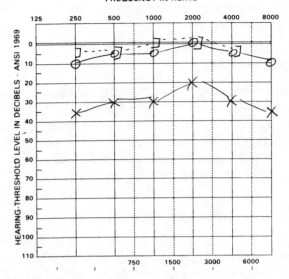

This example of an audiogram shows normal hearing in the right ear (as depicted by the circles) and a 20 dB hearing loss in the left ear (as depicted by the X's). The symbol "]" symbolizes a bone conduction hearing threshold for the right ear.

couraged. For instance, when the child hears a tone, he is instructed to put a block in the box. The audiologist praises him and encourages him to repeat the behavior until he learns (or is "conditioned") to put a block in the box every time he hears a tone.

The subjective tests for the preschooler are similar to the ones described for the younger child, but now the child is able to cooperate verbally. For the first test, the child is asked to repeat the words that the audiologist says over the speakers (such as hot dog, cowboy, ice cream) until he can no longer hear them. Then the audiologist "plays" with him, by asking him to perform a task at the sound of a tone, both with earphones on and without earphones on. Finally, she tests the child with the tympanometer.

If this sequence is unsuccessful with a child in this age range, the audiologist usually resorts to the testing used with a younger child.

The Child Over Age 5

The older child is tested with standard audiometry procedures: that is, he is instructed to raise his hand whenever he hears a tone through the earphone, and repeat the word the audiologist says. Another test that may be introduced at this time (or even with a younger, cooperative child) will evaluate the child's speech-sound discrimination.

What Has the Audiologist Learned?

In a relatively short period (30 minutes to an hour), the audiologist has learned not only about your child's hearing, but also about his overall personality. In testing his hearing ability,

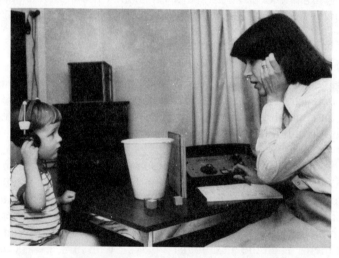

Children learn to play "games" with the audiologist, who measures the child's hearing by teaching them to drop a block in the box at the sound of the tone. *(Photo by Jerry A. McCoy)*

the audiologist has determined if there is a hearing impairment, how much and what kind of a hearing loss is present and which ear is affected. She has learned if the child responds appropriately to a social situation and she has made some observations about his intellectual and neuromuscular development.

How Can a Hearing Evaluation Be Accurate Despite a Child's Lack of Cooperation?

Some parents may doubt the accuracy of an audiologist's evaluation of their child's hearing. A child may be grouchy, tired or in discomfort because of ear pain, rendering him uncooperative. Or, the child may be in a rambunctious or "eager beaver" mood, and all too willing to keep dropping blocks into the box even if he doesn't hear the tone! At the end of a testing session, an exasperated parent of a 3-year-old may look at the test results and doubt their validity. How could the scores be accurate when my child behaved in such an uncooperative manner?

However, audiologists trained to work with children are faced daily with tired, irritable, uncooperative, restless, or overeager children. They keenly observe the child's behavior, shape it, and factor it into their evaluation of the child's reactions.

Throughout the testing, the audiologist has certain reliability checks to tell her if she is assessing the child's hearing accurately. She is watching your child every second for clues that will give her insight into his hearing. One reason why the audiologist performs so many different tests is that she can never rely on only one test result to make her assessment: two of three tests must agree in order to determine her final impression.

In fact, much of the behavior your child exhibits throughout the testing may provide clues to hearing problems. Even a crying baby can be tested in some situations; for example, the audiologist may notice a pause or change in the crying when the child hears a sound. Often, a child who has just fallen asleep can be tested because he responds to sounds at the beginning of his sleep state.

Again, an audiologist specifically trained to work with children is best able to make these judgments and assess your child's behavior.

SPEECH-LANGUAGE PATHOLOGIST: DETECTING LEVEL OF LANGUAGE

Learning a language is like building a tower of blocks: each block must be placed carefully on top of the other, and if one block is missing, succeeding blocks have no foundation. Like the tower, your child's language development progresses in phases. With each learned phase, the child is ready to proceed to the next step. If any phase is incomplete or missing, the foundation of his language may be weak enough to affect other skills, such as reading and writing.

Parents often are unaware of the fact that there are different definitions for speech and language. Language is a code we learn to communicate ideas, and includes reading, writing, gesturing and speaking. Speech is the spoken form of language. Articulation is the process by which sounds, syllables

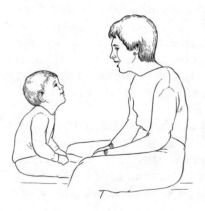

If a parent is aware that a child is not hearing well because of middle ear fluid, she can spend extra time emphasizing speech and playing word games with the child to help compensate for speech that the child may not be hearing.

and words are formed when your tongue, jaw, teeth, lips and palate alter the air stream coming from the vocal folds.

If your child has suffered mild to moderate hearing loss over many months due to persistent or intermittent middle ear fluid, his speech-language abilities may be below normal limits for a child his age. As a parent, you can detect difficulties in speech and language in the following ways:

If the child does not meet the milestones for speech and language at appropriate times as described in the chart at the end of the chapter.

Any change in your child's speech and language can signal a hearing loss. For instance, you may suspect a hearing loss if your child's speech and language has been progressing normally, but suddenly stops improving or seems to regress.

Observe your child's interactions with his friends. Is he able to communicate with them? Are his verbal skills comparable?

When your child's hearing is being tested by an audiologist skilled in working with children, ask her to screen your child's speech and language ability.

One mother, whose daughter suffered a hearing loss because of persistent middle ear fluid, said: "Beth had started talking very early and her pronunciation had always been good. All of a sudden, she wasn't pronouncing as well and I noticed she wasn't hearing me. It's hard to tell when you have a two-and-one-half-year old if she's deliberately ignoring you. But there were times when I would be standing right behind her and say, 'Would you like a piece of candy?' and she didn't even respond."

If you have been referred to a speech-language pathologist (SLP), or if you believe your child needs to be evaluated, it's best to find a SLP trained in working with children. The SLP is trained to identify specific problem areas in speech and language and to determine the direction for therapy to correct the problems. The SLP should be certified by the American Speech and Hearing Association and/or should be licensed by the state in which she works, if licensing is required.

The SLP will test the child for pronunciation of words, his

functional use of language (such as syntax and grammar), his understanding of language and how he expresses himself. She will test his voice quality and the rate at which he talks. Like the audiologist, the SLP is trained to evaluate your child's social and emotional behavior and may spend time "playing" with the child or watching him interact with a parent, siblings, or other children in the waiting room. These observations will give her clues about underlying problems of speech and language.

THE TEACHER: ASKING FOR SPECIAL ATTENTION IN THE CLASSROOM

The pupil who has a hearing loss may be perceived by a teacher as inattentive, meddlesome, hyperactive or uncooperative. If the child cannot hear what the teacher is saying, he may get up and wander to the back of the room to study a science display or look out the window. If the child cannot hear well enough to understand instructions, he may look at another child's paper. If the child has not heard his name being called, he will not respond.

If your child is experiencing intermittent hearing loss, you should speak personally with your child's teacher to explain the situation. The teacher is then able to understand your child's behavior, and to use common-sense remedies. For example, she can seat your child at the front of the class and away from distracting noises, such as an air conditioner, heater, or aquarium. If one ear has better hearing than the other, then the child should be seated with the good ear nearer the teacher. Many teachers are very aware of intermittent hearing loss in children under the age of 10 and make it a point to always speak facing the children (instead of at the blackboard) since visual clues are very important for children with hearing loss.

As another way to be on guard against undetected hearing loss, ask the teacher to call you if the child acts particularly hard of hearing or if his behavior changes dramatically. Additionally, periodic talks with the teacher may be helpful to discuss your child's educational progress and assess whether your child's development is comparable to his peers. Even if your child lags behind the other children for a season because of hearing loss, it will be very easy for him to catch up academically once his hearing improves. In some cases, however, he may need some help, such as tutoring.

NOTES

1. Downs M, Blager FB. The Otitis Prone Child. Developmental and Behavioral Pediatrics. 1982 June: 3(2).
2. Northern JL, Downs M. Hearing in Children. 1975: Williams and Wilkins.
3. Personal Communication. Robert Wood Johnson Foundation Program Summary. Grant numbers 8553, 8556, 8543, 8557, 8561.

SPEECH AND LANGUAGE SCREENING QUESTIONNAIRE

Age 3 Months to 5 Months

_____ Is baby quieted by familiar voice?

_____ Does baby respond to talking by looking at speaker?

_____ Does baby respond to sounds by quieting?

_____ Does baby have a special cry for hunger?

_____ Does baby make vocal sound when played with?

_____ Does baby connect two syllables when vocalizing?

Age 6 Months to 8 Months

_____ Does baby respond to angry or friendly voices differently?

_____ Does baby look around to locate person talking?

_____ Does baby respond to name by stopping and listening?

_____ Can baby produce 4 or 5 sounds in a chain?

_____ Is baby beginning to make sounds for pleasure?

_____ Is baby beginning to make sounds when playing with toys?

Age 9 Months to 11 Months

_____ Does child stop activity at hearing noise?

_____ Is child beginning to enjoy looking at pictures when they are named?

_____ Will child respond with gestures to some words? (Waves when you say "bye-bye," lifts arms when you say "come" or "up"?)

_____ Does child enjoy imitating sounds like tongue click or "horsey gallop"?

_____ Does child play games like "peek-a-boo" or "patty-cake"?

_____ Does child copy melody pattern of familiar phrases, such as "thank you," "up-we-go"?

Age 12 Months to 17 Months

_____ Does child enjoy listening to speakers?

_____ Will child look at ball when asked: "Where is ball?"

_____ Will child look at mom or dad when asked: "Where is mamma?"; "Where is daddy?"

_____ Does child say first real words, such as "mama," "da da," "bye-bye"?

_____ Does child use voice and gesture to obtain a wanted object?

_____ Does child use jargon of sentence-like sounds when playing, with sometimes a real word coming in?

Age 18 Months to 23 Months

_____ Will child point to picture or familiar objects when named, like doggie

_____ Will child bring something from another room if asked?

_____ Can child point to one or more body parts on self, or on a doll?

_____ Does child use real words and fewer gestures when trying to get something?

_____ Can child name one picture of a familiar object?

_____ Does child use 10 words with meaning?

Age 24 Months to 29 Months

_____ Can child follow two simple commands with same object? "Get the book and give it to me," or "Get the car, and put it on the table."

_____ Can child follow directions with one preposition (in, on)?

_____ Can child point to four body parts?

_____ Does child combine two words in sequence? (car go)

_____ Does child refer to self by using name?

_____ Does child have a vocabulary of 20 words, used with meaning?

Age 30 Months to 35 Months

_____ Does child understand "action words," and will child point to one or two pictures of someone sleeping, playing, sitting, pulling, etc.?

_____ Can child point to 10 pictures of everyday objects when you name them? (house, dog, shoe, cup, baby, etc.)

_____ Can child follow directions with two prepositions?

_____ Can child name one color correctly?

_____ Does child use three words in sequence? (see car go)

_____ Can child name five pictures of familiar objects?

Age 36 Months to 47 Months

_____ Does child follow directions with two or three prepositions? (in, on, under, behind, in front)

_____ Can child point to pictures of action words? (playing, sleeping, washing)

_____ Can child follow three simple directions with same objects? "Get the car, put it on the table and sit down."

_____ Can child recite a four-line nursery rhyme song?

_____ Does child use three-word sentences?

_____ Can child give full name?

Age 45 Months to 59 Months

_____ Can child follow directions with four prepositions?

_____ Can child follow three unrelated commands? ("Put the book on your lap, clap your hands and give me the paper.")

_____ Can child correctly point to many familiar objects? (20 to 30)

_____ Can child count three objects?

_____ Does child use four-word sentences?

_____ Can child answer questions about what you do when "hungry" or "hurt yourself"?

Age 60 Months and Over

_____ Can child give right hand upon request?

_____ Can child select an item that is heavier from one that is lighter?

_____ Can child understand most of what you say to him?

_____ Can child define and describe use of four common words? (shoe, book, house, hat)

_____ Can child give his age?

_____ Can child name three coins?

From Speech and Language Screening Questionnaire, Experimental Edition, © 1981 by Florence Berman Blazer, Ph.D., University of Colorado Health Sciences Center, Denver, Colorado.

CHAPTER FOUR

Treatment

Most often, otitis media is treated to kill bacteria that is causing symptoms of pain and fever, to prevent structural damage to the eardrum and middle ear, to equalize air pressure in the middle ear and to ventilate a middle ear that is filled with fluid (specific treatments for these conditions are discussed in Part Two, Chapter 2). Although hearing loss can accompany any of these abnormal conditions, hearing is usually restored once an abnormal middle ear condition is effectively treated.

Occasionally, persistent middle ear fluid will cause no symptoms of pain or discomfort and will pose little or no threat to damaging the eardrum or middle ear structures. In these instances, however, the primary concern of the parents and the physician is that the child is suffering a hearing loss likely to result in delayed speech or language development. If the child is tested and found to be suffering a significant hearing loss and is lagging in speech development, the parent and physician may discuss the following treatments to restore hearing to normal levels.

TREATMENT: SURGICAL INTERVENTION

Few, if any, treatment decisions in pediatric practice are made more often, and entail more uncertainties, than decisions about tympanostomy tube placement for otitis media . . . The main concerns are usually not about symptoms . . . but rather about long-term effects, namely middle ear damage or impaired speech, language or intellectual development. These concerns must, on the other hand, be weighed against the liability of secretory otitis media and its tendency to eventually resolve spontaneously, the cost, risks and sequelae of tube placement and the absence, after all, of convincing evidence linking otitis media early in life to either otologic or developmental difficulties later in life.[1]

If medication fails to clear middle ear fluid and hearing loss persists, then insertion of tympanostomy tubes may be advised to restore hearing. The decision to subject a child to surgery should be considered carefully and should not be made until the child's condition has been monitored for several months (See Part Four). If you doubt the rationale for a treatment plan suggested for your child, do not hesitate to seek the professional opinion of several specialists. In fact, many insurance companies require a second opinion before they will reimburse surgery costs.

Some experts advise parents against blithely accepting excessive treatment for their children to prevent speech and language development delays. Dr. Paradise warns: "We should not submit large numbers of children to surgical intervention early in the course of their (ear) illnesses because of fear of later developmental handicaps. This risks more harm than good."[2]

Most parents have difficulty determining whether or not their children should have an operation, such as insertion of tympanostomy tubes, to preserve or restore normal hearing. To help sort out this dilemma, a comparison can be drawn showing how a different type of surgeon approaches a similar problem.

The orthopedic surgeon operates on bones and joints. If a patient has suffered repeated injury to a knee joint, for example, the orthopedic surgeon will carefully examine the knee using X-rays and special tests. The surgeon may then recommend surgery to preserve the knee's normal function and to prevent further damage that could lead to impaired function. A parent might question the surgeon: "If my child does not have knee surgery, would that mean that he might not be able to walk?" The surgeon would probably reply that the child's ability to walk is not really at risk. Rather it might mean the child would be unable to participate in sports and could predispose him to development of knee ailments during adult life.

Similarly, a parent may over-simplify the decision of ear surgery by asking: "Without the ear operation, will my child go deaf?" The ear surgeon's answer will invariably be, "No." But when dealing with middle ear surgery, including insertion of tympanostomy tubes, total deafness is really not the issue. The issue is whether or not the ear surgeon should intervene in order to restore or preserve normal middle ear function. The orthopedic surgeon knows when to recommend that a knee needs surgery, and an ear surgeon has been fully trained to know when surgery is needed to maintain or preserve normal hearing in the ear.

TREATMENT: SPEECH THERAPY ━━━━━

If the child is shown to have a speech-language delay by a speech-language pathologist (SLP), the SLP may suggest a program in which the child works with the SLP several times a week and at home with his parents.

Marion Downs, MA, DHS, has studied the relationship between intermittent hearing loss and speech delays. She suggests that a language screening test should be done if the child suffers three consecutive months of middle ear fluid. If the child has any language delays, an at-home stimulation program could help the child with language.[3] These measures have resulted in marked gains in performance of children who were showing problems with language acquisition.

TREATMENT: HEARING AIDS ═══════════

Hearing aids are rarely needed for children who suffer intermittent hearing loss as a result of persistent middle ear fluid. Most children are able to compensate for short periods of hearing loss by reading lips, moving closer to the speaker or asking the speaker to talk louder. They also are usually able to "catch up" on any missed speech development once the fluid has cleared from their ears.

However, some children with persistent middle ear fluid may benefit from the use of a hearing aid. Again, the child's lifestyle must be taken into consideration. For instance, a child with a below normal intelligence who needs all the hearing he can get in every situation may be fitted for a hearing aid, even if his loss is classified as mild. Conversely, a hearing aid may be unnecessary for a child with a hearing loss of 25 dB who is of superior intelligence and has developed good listening skills.

Some children may be candidates for hearing aids, even when hearing loss is intermittent, if speech, language and educational performance has been affected. For example, a child who has suffered chronic middle ear fluid from infancy and who has not responded well to antimicrobial treatment or the insertion of tympanostomy tubes may benefit from a hearing aid. This child may suffer a hearing loss of 30 to 40 dB for many months out of the year.[4]

Why couldn't a child be fitted with a hearing aid instead of having tympanostomy tubes inserted? First, tympanostomy tubes are inserted to correct a condition in the middle ear that may cause structural damage and result in serious problems. Second, a hearing aid can be a difficult object for a preschooler or school-aged child to contend with. And in many cases, parents, doctors and audiologists may decide against the hearing aid because they believe the child may not cooperate in wearing or learning to use the aid.

FOLLOW-UP TREATMENT

A child who has had significant hearing loss from otitis media should have periodic follow-up medical examinations and hearing tests. These measures will give the physician or speech-language pathologist a chance to adjust treatment if hearing improves or worsens. For instance, if a child is on prophylactic antibiotics and his hearing has been normal for five months during the winter season, the physician may decide to discontinue medication.

Once the child's hearing returns to normal and the middle ear condition has cleared up, regular examination is unnecessary unless the parent detects a recurrence of hearing loss.

QUESTIONS AND ANSWERS

Q: At what point will a child with middle ear fluid experience hearing loss?

A: Almost all children with middle ear fluid experience some hearing loss. On a daily basis you will not know to what degree your child is experiencing hearing loss. In general, you should not worry about the intermittent hearing loss that your child may experience with middle ear fluid. However, if your child has a history *of recurrent ear infections and middle ear fluid, it is wise to monitor hearing, speech-language development and educational achievement, especially at times when you suspect a hearing loss.*

Q: Although I sense my daughter is suffering some hearing loss, I can't be sure about it. She is at an age when she becomes preoccupied with play, and at other times she may simply ignore me. How can I tell if it's her hearing or if she's just ignoring me?

A: If your child is two-and-one-half years or older, here is a simple word game that you can use at home to detect a hearing loss. Sit down on the floor with your child facing you, and place five familiar objects or pictures of objects in front of her, each of which have two syllables in their names, such as cowboy, hot dog or ice cream. Call out each object's name in a normal conversational tone and ask her to point to the one you call out. Praise her for her success, and then say you're going to play the game again. This time, put your hand over your mouth and repeat the exercise. A third time, put your hand over your mouth and whisper the names of the objects. A child should be able to hear even the whisper.

The purpose of this admittedly crude form of testing is to assure many parents that their child's hearing is close to normal. But it does not take the place of professional testing by a specialist, such as an audiologist, who is trained to work with children. If your child does not perform well on the test above and/or if you continue to suspect a hearing loss, it's best to follow your instincts and have the child's hearing tested.

NOTES

1. Paradise JL, Rogers K. On Otitis Media, Child Development and Tympanostomy Tubes: New Answers or Old Questions? Pediatrics 1986 Jan: 77(1):88–92.
2. Paradise JL. Otitis Media during Early Life: How Hazardous to Development? Pediatrics 1981 Dec: 68(6): 867–73.
3. Downs M. "Audiologist's Overview of Sequelae of Early Otitis Media" in Workshop on Effects of Otitis Media on Children. Pediatrics. 1983 April:71(4):643.
4. Northern JL, Downs M. Hearing in Children. 1975: Williams and Wilkins.

PART SEVEN

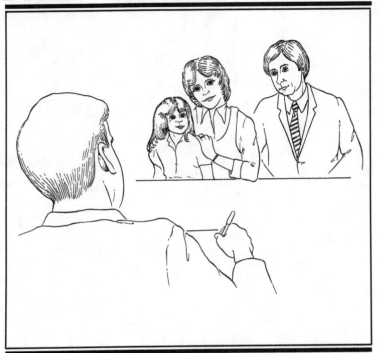

The Parent and Physician as a Team

The Parent
and Physician
as a Team

I. THE PARENT AS PART
OF THE MEDICAL TEAM

As the price of medical care soars, patients are becoming discerning consumers as they search for the best treatment at the most reasonable prices. At the same time, they are becoming educated consumers as the mass media—TV, newspapers, magazines, self-help books—brings a greater understanding of medical science into the household. As a result, many parents are now taking an active role in their child's health care by exercising preventive measures and by asking questions of their child's doctor.

Achieving a good working relationship with a doctor can be a difficult task, particularly when your child suffers repeated ear infections. Many parents do not understand the disease or a doctor's reasons for treatment or methods of management. They may blame the doctor for the problem's recurrence, or they may become resentful of the constant medications and office visits required to treat the ear infection. Rather than vent their frustrations, many parents will change pediatricians.

Seeking answers to the causes and prevention of your child's otitis media may seem a lot like detective work, but it will be easier if you and your physician form a working relationship. The physician who uses respect and consideration in dealing with a parent and child is building a foundation of a long-lasting, beneficial relationship. At the same time, the parent who is honest, inquisitive and informed can add a further dimension to the relationship. As trust builds, the physician will be more willing to include a parent in the decision-making process, and the parent will be more likely to trust a physician's advice.

This relationship can be especially valuable to the parent in times of stress. No matter how educated or sophisticated parents may be, a child's illness may cause them to lean on a physician for emotional support. A frightened and anxious parent is seeking authoritative answers from a trusted person and if a trust has already been established, the crisis may be resolved much faster.

HOW PARENTS CAN HELP THEIR DOCTORS

Your Relationship With Your Doctor

Many patients are intimidated by their doctor, and consequently are afraid to ask questions or offer comments and suggestions. Why do we feel this way about doctors? As one doctor put it: "The patient needs to feel the doctor is trustworthy, and one way the physician makes the patient feel that is to use an authoritarian approach. It's hard to question authority. It's really tough for people to be critical of people on whom they're dependent."[1]

By remaining silent, parents are missing a chance to develop a healthy parent-physician relationship. By simply nodding their heads in silent agreement, parents are telling the physician they understand and agree with his explanations—even if they didn't comprehend a word he said. By not verbalizing feelings or asking questions, parents are creating a situation in which anger, frustration, resentment and skepticism can build in the relationship.

The longer parents remain silent, the harder it is to change the pattern of the parent-doctor relationship. Many parents would rather switch doctors than ask questions or challenge a doctor about treatment. However, had these parents opened up, they might have been surprised at the receptiveness extended by the physician. As one parent said: "You have to trust in your pediatrician or you'd be lost, but you also have to use your own intuition."

How can you establish a better give-and-take interaction with your physician?

First, parents must understand that no single treatment method is always effective for all children. Doctors have more than one treatment option—and this holds true for parents. Rather than passively "taking orders" from a physician, parents can ask questions, learn and seek information, without being adversarial. If you have not developed this type of working relationship with your child's doctor, then start by taking these steps:

- Let your doctor know that you want to take a more active role and participate in decisions.

- Make sure that you always understand what your child's doctor is telling you about your child's condition.

- If you are not sure what your child's doctor is doing or saying, ask questions.

- When a doctor prescribes medication, advises consultation with a specialist or recommends surgery, ask why that particular choice has been made and ask what the alternatives are.

- If you question the propriety of the treatment, seek additional information before proceeding. Only on rare occasions, such as when there is a serious complication present, is it necessary to make a decision rapidly. Usually, there is time for you to gain full understanding of the situation, to learn about and consider alternatives, and to seek second medical opinions. Never feel "dumb" because the physician has to explain something to you several times before you are able to comprehend it; nor should you ever feel guilty for requesting an explanation about a treatment that has been advised.

If it's hard for you to question your doctor in person—or if your child is crying and you'd like to get home immediately—think about your questions and write them down. Call the office and tell the nurse or receptionist that you would like your doctor to return your call. After several phone conversations, you'll find it easier to ask your doctor questions in his office.

One factor that discourages parents from talking to their doctors is the hurried environment associated with a doctor's office. When a patient has waited for an hour to see a doctor, and knows there are other ill children in the waiting room, the parent may feel guilty about taking too much of the physician's time. In this situation, the parent may ask the physician to call her back later in the day after the doctor has finished seeing patients.

Collecting Information

Carolyn sat nervously tapping on the chair in the doctor's office as she held her son Michael in her lap. She had been referred to an ENT specialist because of Michael's recurrent ear infections, and was nervous and anxious about what the specialist would find in her child's ears and she was frightened that surgery might be needed.

The specialist set Carolyn at ease by introducing himself and asking her about Michael and his interests and development. But she began to feel some tension as the specialist began to discuss Michael's ear infections.

"Since I didn't receive a summary of Michael's problems from your pediatrician, I'd like to ask you some

questions about Michael's experiences with ear infec-
tions," began the specialist.

Carolyn could answer some of the questions, but she
realized she was omitting some very important infor-
mation. The specialist asked her questions such as: When
did the ear infections begin? What are his symptoms?
How many has he had? Which ear has been infected the
greater number of times? What medications does he take,
and for how long, has he been taking them?

At the end of the consultation, Carolyn felt pleased
with the specialist's thorough examination and diagnosis.
However, she called the pediatrician's office that after-
noon to collect additional information about her son's
ear infections to be better prepared to answer questions
on her next visit to the specialist.

This story illustrates a common breakdown in communication. Your child's doctor formulates a diagnosis based on
information obtained from you, and from results of any additional X-ray or laboratory tests. But without this information,
the ear specialist is restricted in his decision-making.

Although some doctors may take a rather casual approach
in collecting information about your child's ear problems, such
an approach is not of maximal benefit to your child; a lack of
precise information can even lead to mishaps or inappropriate
treatment. For example, you may tell a doctor that you are
concerned about the frequent infections that your child has
had and about the amount of medication he has been given
for ear infections. When you bring these concerns to the attention of a doctor, he should take the time to thoroughly
review your child's problems with ear infections and the resultant treatment.

On the next page is a form that parents can use in keeping
track of their child's condition to help both pediatrician and
specialist to understand your child's ear problems and aid in
providing accurate information in making a proper diagnosis.

Otitis Media Data Sheet

DATE:

Right Ear
Left Ear

SYMPTOMS:

MEDICATION (include specific kind and duration):

Pain Relievers:
Decongestants/Antihistamines:
Antibiotics:
Other:

OTHER TREATMENT:

Myringotomy
Tympanocentesis (and results):
Forcible inflation of middle ear:
Other:

REASON FOR DOCTOR'S VISIT
(include doctor's diagnosis):

Acute visit:
Follow-up Visit:
Well-baby Visit:

HEARING ABILITY:

Seems normal
Possibly impaired, explain:
Test results

SPEECH DEVELOPMENT:

Too young to assess
Seems normal
Seems the child's vocabulary lags behind peers
Test results:

Preparing Your Child for Office Visits

Few children enjoy the experience of having a physician "poking" around in their ears with a strange-looking instrument. Some babies and children will scream, cry and try to wriggle away in spite of all measures to prepare them beforehand or to make them comfortable during the procedure. In fact, parents can expect this reaction from most children and shouldn't feel their child is any worse than any other who will be examined by the physician. The physician also expects and is prepared for this reaction.

Although the parent and doctor may not be able to prevent an unhappy reaction, prior preparation and a gentle approach may lessen the older child's fears and may make a baby less anxious.

Since a baby cannot be prepared beforehand for an office visit, it's up to the physician to approach the baby in a gentle and unhurried manner. For instance, the baby can be allowed to touch the otoscope and the physician can do some playacting with the parent and let the baby watch as the physician examines the parent's ears.

These measures can also work miracles with an older child who may be very curious about the otoscope and who would be delighted to try to "blow out" the light on the instrument. However, older children can also be prepared even before they enter the doctor's office by parents who discuss the reasons for the examination, how the examination will be performed and what the doctor will do during the visit. Some books that can help a child prepare for a doctor's visit include: *The Berenstain Bears Go to the Doctor,* by Stan and Jan Berenstain, Random House, 1981; *The Checkup,* by Helen Oxbury, Dial Books, 1983; and *My Doctor,* by Harlow Rockwell, MacMillan, 1973.

How can the behavior of a parent during an examination affect the behavior of a child? Obviously, any parent is going to become tense when their child starts to scream and yell at the touch of an examining instrument. Words of encouragement and comfort from a parent may not stop the unhappy

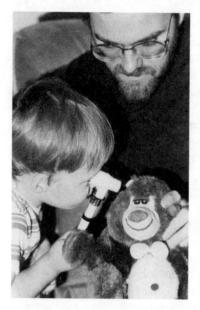

Many children will be less frightened of the ear examination if they are familiar with the instruments and can discuss their upcoming doctor's visit with their parents. Here, a child plays doctor with his teddy bear by examining the bear's ears with an earscope. *(Photo by Cynthia J. Carney)*

reaction, but they can at least be reassuring to the child through her tears. On the other hand, a child's unhappy reaction may get worse if a parent gets angry and yells at the child to be quiet, or even threatens to slap the child. A child should not be told he is "bad" or "wrong," nor should he be ridiculed because of his fears.

Sometimes, you may want to ask your doctor to end the examination if your child is becoming hysterical. It may be better to just admit the examination is not going well and discuss with your doctor other approaches to make your child more comfortable and less fearful. Unless it is suspected that your child has a serious condition that needs immediate treatment, end the examination and try again a day or two later with a different approach. In the long term, it is better to establish a good doctor-child relationship than to overpower an uncooperative, fearful child who will subsequently be more reluctant to return to the doctor's office for further care.

II. WHAT TO EXPECT FROM THE PRIMARY CARE PHYSICIAN

The pediatrician or family physician is the first link in the chain of medical caretakers who will be treating your child's ear problems. The primary care physician has the responsibility of examining and diagnosing your child's acute ear infections (discussed in Part One, Chapter 4) and monitoring the condition. Ultimately, your child will either outgrow the ear infections or your child's primary care physician may recommend a specialist if he believes surgery is indicated.

How Pediatricians and Family Physicians Are Trained

Pediatricians attend four years of college and four years of medical school before entering a three-year pediatric residency training program. Throughout that program, pediatric residents work in hospitals and clinics caring for ill children and "rotate" through different departments of the hospital to gain a generalized education of the various medical specialties. Pediatricians may elect to be certified by the American Board of Pediatrics by passing written and oral examinations and successfully completing three years of hospital-based training in general pediatrics.

Family physicians also complete the same number of years in education; however, their residency program takes place in a family practice center which gives the residents first-hand experience working as a family physician. Six areas in which the physicians concentrate are internal medicine, pediatrics, obstetrics-gynecology, psychology and neurology, surgical workup and community medicine. Ambulatory care is a focus during their residency training. Family physicians may elect to become certified by the American Board of Family Practice by completing residency training and successfully passing a two-day written examination. This certification must be renewed every seven years.

Role of the Primary Care Physician

Diagnosis.   The pediatrician or family physician looks, at many ears. The most frequent type of visit to pediatricians is for well-baby and well-child care; the second most common reason for visiting a pediatrician is for management of otitis media.[2] A busy pediatrician who sees about 30 patients a day has an average of 15 to 20 minutes to spend with each child. In this time, he must be able to adequately visualize the eardrum and make a diagnosis.

As discussed in Part One, Chapter 4, physicians have a responsibility to thoroughly examine a child's ears, even if that means cleaning out wax, talking with the child beforehand to allay fears or struggling with an uncooperative child. Many parents prefer a short period of unhappiness for their child in exchange for a thorough examination and diagnosis in which they feel confident. Parents who detect a hurried and incomplete examination may not be convinced their child received the best treatment.

Follow-Up Visits.   Routine follow-up examination after a bout of acute otitis media is widely recommended in medical textbooks to determine if the infection has cleared and if there is any fluid left in the ear that could interfere with hearing. Some pediatricians schedule follow-up visits two weeks after a child has had an ear infection; others postpone the visit for six to eight weeks.

Recently, the value of follow-up visits in treating acute otitis media has been questioned. Studies show a child's eardrum

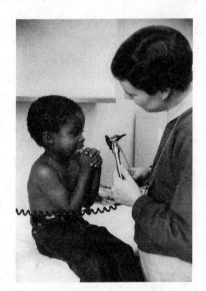

Physicians who approach a child gently and cautiously with an otoscope are more likely to establish a trusting relationship with the child. Here, a physician lets the child look at the otoscope and become familiar with it before she uses it to examine the child's ears. *(Photo courtesy of the Association for the Care of Children's Health)*

may take up to three months to return to its normal appearance,[3] and most children have fluid remaining in the ear two weeks after an ear infection.[4] Even 48 hours after the acute symptoms of an ear infection have cleared, fluid can sometimes be seen bulging against a discolored eardrum.

Therefore, a child does not necessarily have to be reexamined by a physician unless the acute symptoms do not subside, or if a hearing loss is noticed. A follow-up visit at 30 to 60 days after acute otitis media is adequate and possibly more reasonable than the traditional "re-check" of the ears after 10 days on antibiotic. Waiting the 30–60 days allows time for the middle ear fluid to resolve and for the eardrum to return to its normal appearance.

Many children are reexamined too often after acute otitis media. One survey estimated that roughly 54 percent of all visits for otitis media in 1985 were for follow-up visits.[5] The very frequent re-check some doctors advise can be costly to the parent both financially and in time lost from work or time the child loses from school (or a daycare or playgroup). More important, many of the medications prescribed because fluid is observed in a child's ear during a "routine 10-day re-check" may be unnecessary.

Ask your doctor why the re-check is necessary. Have him explain exactly what he is looking for and expects to find upon reexamination. If your child's doctor wants to prescribe a second antibiotic even though your child seems to have recovered completely, then ask the doctor to explain what his reasons are. If the doctor tells you that the second antibiotic is needed to help "clear up the fluid," ask him to explain further the scientific evidence for this medical advice.

Physicians at the University of North Carolina Medical School evaluated their rationale for follow-up visits when they noticed many parents did not return for appointments after episodes of otitis media. In reviewing studies that indicate that results of otoscopic examinations are likely to remain abnormal for months after the initial diagnosis, they concluded that a re-check within the first three weeks of an ear infection "may be of marginal value."[6]

Be careful about having your child examined too frequently and given too much antibiotics for otitis media. Make sure you understand and are comfortable with the care your child is receiving.

Monitoring the Child's Condition

It is the end of the month, and John and Carolyn are reviewing their expenses, their insurance records and their bank statements. "Look at this, Carolyn," says John as he begins to add up the figures. "We were reimbursed $120 in office visits and $60 for medications in the past three months. What's going on here? I didn't realize (daughter) Susan was going to the doctor that much!"

Carolyn leans over and starts going through the rec-
ords. She looks at John and shakes her head. "I can't
believe this. I know Susan's been sick a lot, but I didn't
realize we've been to the doctor this many times. I guess
I just haven't been keeping track."

They begin to talk about other consequences of Susan's
illnesses—sleepless nights, cancelled appointments, missed
work, constant medication. All of a sudden, it dawns on
them that their daughter must have a serious problem.
They decide to make an appointment with their pediatri-
cian to discuss the condition and determine if Susan's ear
problems could be managed in a less costly and time-
consuming manner.

The cumulative effects of a child's medical condition can
slowly "creep up" on a family until the parents sit back and
review of the situation. Often, this is a jolting realization that
causes much consternation among parents: Why didn't we
notice that this was happening? Is my child really ill? Have
we waited too long to do something about it?

Often, a pediatrician or family doctor can prevent this situation by reviewing the child's condition with the parents
during every visit. Although two or three ear infections during
a winter season is no cause for alarm, a pediatrician should
take note of a child who seems to constantly suffer from ear
infections. As a pattern of frequent ear infections emerges,
the physician and parent can discuss methods for alleviating
and preventing the episodes. This way, both the parent and
physician are keeping track of the condition and evaluating it
as it happens, instead of waiting until the condition is chronic.

Similarly, the pediatrician can put into perspective a child's
illness. Some parents whose children suffer recurrent ear infections become obsessed with the condition. They feel guilty
and helpless because they can't prevent the infections, and
view their child as "ill." In this situation, pediatricians can
point out that most children under the age of 5 suffer three to
four infections in a winter, as well as five colds per year.[7] If

parents know that their child's illnesses fall within normal ranges, their fears and anxieties may be eased.

The Pediatrician or Family Physician as a Teacher. One pediatrician commented: "The biggest problem with many parents is they have no idea what otitis media is—and most people just don't say anything to us because they don't understand what we're talking about."

The primary care physician can take steps to educate parents about ear infections. Many parents hold misconceptions about otitis media and greatly fear harmful effects from ear infections.

What can physicians do to educate their patients about otitis media even before the patient's first ear infection? Many pediatricians give hand-outs to new patients, such as information about office hours, when to call the office, tips about nursing. Included in these hand-outs could be some literature about otitis media—definitions of ear infections, the difference between an acute ear infection and middle ear fluid, signs and symptoms of ear infections, what to do when your sick child awakens at night with a suspected ear infection, when to call the doctor. One group of Washington, D.C., pediatricians give a "patient information bulletin" which discusses the frequency of ear infections, the methods of diagnosis, the reason for antibiotics and side effects of antibiotics.

One pediatrician from the University of Texas Health Science Center at Dallas Southwestern Medical School says parental education about otitis media is "particularly important if the episode of disease is the child's first."[8] Charles M. Ginsburg, M.D., in a paper presented to a symposium on pediatric patient education, further states that this information should include: (1) a perspective on the problem—is it "normal" for children to get ear infections?, (2) an explanation of the ear's anatomy, (3) symptoms such as pain and hearing loss, (4) a discussion of medications and how they should be administered, (5) potential side effects of the medications, (6) when and how the child should be expected to improve, (7) whether any limitations should be imposed on the child, and (8) a discussion of follow-up visits.

Although preprinted information, videotaped material and education by nurses or physician's assistants can be used in educating the parent, Dr. Ginsburg says: "It's imperative that the initial communication with the parents originate with the physician."

When a child's ear infections become recurrent, and the primary care physician refers the child to an ENT specialist, the physician should prepare the parents for the visit to the specialist. Many parents may become concerned and anxious because their child needs to see a specialist. Their fears may be allayed if the pediatrician (1) explains the reasons for the need of a visit to a specialist, (2) discusses what conditions the specialist will search for, (3) prepares the parents for questions the specialist will ask, and (4) discusses treatment the specialist may consider.

The Pediatrician as Counselor.   When discussing the causes for recurrent otitis media, a pediatrician may often ask the parents about their personal lives: Is the child in day care? Are there problems in the marriage? Have there been any recent events that might have put the child in an unusually stressful situation, such as a death in the family? Such stress upon a child often leads to a breakdown in the child's immune system if the child becomes fatigued or is not getting proper nutrition.

However, a pediatrician who puts too much emphasis on stress as a possible reason for ear infections may be ignoring other physical problems. One parent said her pediatrician was sure that the child was suffering recurrent ear infections because of stress in the home life:

"Our pediatrician thought she wouldn't be getting sick so often if I wasn't working and if she wasn't an only child. I told him I didn't think Heather was waking up at night to get back at us. I thought she was in pain. But he said this behavior was symptomatic of a depressed

child who couldn't deal with her problems in any other way and wants to be reassured that mommy and daddy are still there.

"In our own case, I thought this didn't ring true," she said. "But for a couple of days my husband and I cross-examined ourselves and felt very guilty. Basically, I sat down and I said to myself, 'You're not stupid. You know your child better than anybody. We have a happy home situation. Granted, we're both working and I'm getting a Ph.D., so there is a stress. But I don't see it as a negative stress.' Whether it was gut reaction or mother's intuition, I just thought my child was suffering ear infections for a physical reason."

This mother finally had her child evaluated by an allergist, who determined the child was allergic to dust and started appropriate treatment immediately. The child's constant runny nose and red eyes cleared up and the number of ear infections decreased.

At the other end of the spectrum are parents who apologize for all aspects of their child's behavior by saying, "She's misbehaving today because of her ears." A pediatrician who puts perspective on the problem of otitis media may show a parent that not all behavior can be "blamed" or attributed to a child's ear problems. A child's behavior should be viewed in the framework of her whole life, and should not be limited to a particular illness.

Referral to an Ear Specialist. If the otitis media recurs, at what point should a parent be referred to an ENT specialist for evaluation? It's usually up to the primary care physician to make that suggestion and many doctors set guidelines to determine when to refer. As a general rule, many primary care physicians consider a referral after a child has had three to four ear infections in two consecutive seasons and/or persistent middle ear fluid lasting 10 weeks in both ears with hearing loss, or fluid in one ear lasting 12 weeks with hearing loss.

Some primary care physicians, however, refuse to refer their patients to an ENT specialist for any reason, maintaining surgery or a consultation is unnecessary. Although there are cases when referral to an ENT specialist is unnecessary, this arbitrary and dogmatic approach is unwise. Referral to an ENT specialist should not be equated with a need for surgery. The ear specialist has training and technical abilities that may be beneficial in diagnosis and management of a child's ear problems.

One parent said that her pediatrician told her it was unnecessary to see an ENT specialist.

"But I finally got to the point where I said, 'This child's ears are my responsibility and the fact that he's having these recurring ear problems just doesn't seem right to me.' My doctor finally said that if it would make me feel better, then I could take Brian to a specialist."

Another parent said her doctor didn't refer her to an ENT specialist, even though she noticed that her son wasn't hearing well and that his speech was not as developed as other children his age. Without a referral from her pediatrician, she finally consulted an ENT specialist—who diagnosed middle ear fluid and who referred the child for hearing tests. The hearing test revealed moderate hearing loss in one ear and borderline normal hearing in the other ear. The specialist anesthetized the child's eardrum and removed the fluid (myringotomy) in his office.

"Within hours, Patrick's hearing was better," said the mother. "Although the procedure needed to be repeated in one ear a few months later, I was still dismayed that our pediatrician was so reluctant to refer Patrick to a specialist. I was disappointed in our pediatrician and I may switch to a different pediatrician."

When a primary care physician refers a child to an ear specialist, he should provide the specialist with a summary of relevant medical data. Usually the primary care physician will call or write the specialist, giving such information as number of prior ear infections, medications with which the child has been treated, and allergies, if any. The more information about your child that the specialist has, the more productive will be the time the specialist spends evaluating your child. In fact, the ability of an ear specialist to arrive at a correct diagnosis depends, in large part, upon accuracy and completeness of information available.

III. FINDING AND WORKING WITH AN ENT SPECIALIST

An otolaryngologist specializes in disorders of the head and neck, especially those related to the ear, nose and throat. Otolaryngology is the abbreviated form of otorhinolaryngology, which derives from the Greek roots of oto (ear), rhino (nose), laryn (throat) and ology (study of).

After completing four years of medical school, otolaryngologists embark on five or more years of specialty training. Otolaryngologists perform a great variety of surgical procedures in the daily treatment of disorders involving the ear, nose, sinuses, pharynx and other related structures in the head and neck. Those specially trained in ear work can restore hearing through microsurgery and recognize abnormal conditions involving the eardrum and middle ear.

The otolaryngologist, as an ear surgeon, should know how to differentiate relatively harmless conditions from abnormalities which require medical or surgical intervention. Even for the experienced otolaryngologist, knowing when to recommend surgical intervention can be extremely difficult. Nevertheless, the otolaryngologist is the medical expert who must be responsible for deciding when a child requires surgery for management of middle ear problems.

When an ENT Specialist is Needed

A pediatrician will usually recommend consultation with an otolaryngologist if your child is suffering frequently occurring acute otitis media or persistent middle ear fluid. Other factors that would indicate a consultation are:

Hearing loss, especially if a child's speech development lags behind peers or the child has many articulation errors.

Need for excessive amounts of medication to control ear infections. Does your doctor have to prescribe different antibiotics because he can't find one that works? Does your child suffer side effects from the antibiotics?

Finding an ENT Specialist

Your pediatrician or family doctor probably will give you the names of several competent local otolaryngologists. In addition, you may want to ask friends whose children have had similar ear problems. In finding a suitable ENT specialist for your child, look for a doctor who likes to work with children and who has a reputation for communicating effectively with parents. In addition, find an ear specialist who can conduct your child's hearing tests in his office or at a conveniently-located facility.

Preparing for the Consultation

Before visiting the otolaryngologist, make sure your physician has supplied him with reasons for the referral, a summary of the child's medical history and any test results that may help the specialist decide a course of treatment. You may also want to write out questions for the specialist.

What to Expect From the Consultation

After the specialist has thoroughly examined your child, he will discuss with you his diagnosis and recommend a plan of management. To reach this decision, the specialist will discuss the following factors: the history of the child's illness, including how many ear infections he's had; symptoms; antibiotics prescribed and his reaction to them; other illnesses; and possible allergies.

You should understand that the ear specialist can choose from many alternative treatments; some involve prescribing medication, others minor types of office surgery, and still others may involve surgery under general anesthesia. Though your primary care physician may have implied the ear specialist will recommend tubes, approach the visit without assuming that surgery is needed. You are bringing your child to the ear specialist to gain the benefit of his experience and specialized training in abnormal ear conditions, and treatment by the specialist does not have to include surgery.

The ear specialist should have a good rapport with your child's primary care doctor. You should expect the specialist to promptly call or send a report to your child's primary care doctor, and for a copy of the report. If there seem to be differences of opinion between your specialist and pediatrician, ask the ear specialist to carefully explain reasons for his recommendation and ask for guidance in choosing among alternatives for management.

Finally, you should never get the feeling that the ear specialist is viewing your child as a "potential surgical case." You should feel that the ear specialist will choose judiciously among many alternatives and not jump quickly to a surgical cure.

When the Parent Is Caught in the Middle

Cheryl was speechless. An ENT specialist had just told her that her son was perfectly fine—he didn't need any medication and he didn't need to be seen again by the specialist.

"What do you mean, there's nothing wrong?" said Cheryl. "I mean . . . I'm glad there's nothing wrong.

But why does my pediatrician keep prescribing antibiotics? And why does he keep telling me my son has ear infections?"

The ENT specialist paused. He decided to ask Cheryl a couple of questions: "Mrs. Cooper, when's the last time you saw your pediatrician?"

"Two weeks ago," she replied.

"Why did you visit him?"

"It was a follow-up visit. My pediatrician always asks to see David two weeks after an acute ear infection," said Cheryl.

"Did your pediatrician prescribe antibiotics at that follow up visit?"

When she answered yes, the specialist had another question: "Was David ill, did he have a fever or was he crying or irritable?"

"Oh, no," Cheryl quickly answered. "He was just fine. But the pediatrician said that the ear infection had never gone away and that he needed more antibiotics."

"Why don't you bring him in to see me the next time he seems to have an ear infection," said the specialist. "There's a possibility that David really doesn't have an acute ear infection at times, but that he just has middle ear fluid. In those cases, I would suggest that no treatment is necessary."

After more discussion, Cheryl thanked the specialist and talked to her husband Paul about the visit. They decided to take the specialist's advice, but they decided to go one step further. David's next follow-up visit was in two weeks. Cheryl would take him to the pediatrician, and then she'd go immediately to the specialist's office and see if the two diagnoses were the same.

On the day of the visits, the pediatrician told Cheryl David's ear infection had "not gone away," and suggested another course of antibiotics. When the ENT specialist looked at David's ears, he said there was some fluid in the ear but that was normal for children within three to four weeks after an acute ear infection.

"Let's not do anything for now," he said. "But let me see him in about two months. If the fluid hasn't gone away by then, we'll discuss what to do next."

Cheryl and Paul were perplexed at the differences in advice. They were angry that their son might have been on many months of antibiotics unnecessarily. Paul was ready to find a new pediatrician; Cheryl wanted to talk the situation over with their current pediatrician.

The next week, both Cheryl and Paul visited the pediatrician and told him about the conflicting diagnoses and asked him how that could be avoided in the future. The pediatrician was silent for a while.

"I'm sorry this situation has happened," he said. "I think we have had a misunderstanding." The pediatrician went on to explain that he uses the term "infection" whenever he observes fluid in a child's middle ear. He said that he usually prescribes antibiotic to treat the "infection" even though he knows that only about one-half of the children with fluid in the ears have harmful bacteria in the fluid. The pediatrician said he had been treating children with ear infections in this way for the past 15 years and no parent had ever really questioned him about the rationale for the treatment. Cheryl asked the pediatrician to discuss with the ear specialist her son's ear infections and devise a plan for management.

Although this story is actually a compilation of accounts provided by parents who shared their experiences in the preparation of this book, it illustrates a most important point. The ear specialist who examines your child may provide a viewpoint that differs from that of your child's primary care physician. This should not alarm or even disappoint you. When your child is referred to a specialist, you are seeking the opinion of a doctor who specializes in ear disorders. If the ear specialist has one opinion and the primary care physician has a markedly different one, then the two physicians should resolve their differences and work out a treatment plan.

The best ear specialists are those who can communicate effectively with a child's primary care physician. You should not be placed in the middle. The ear specialist's job is not completed until the primary care physician has been informed of all findings and the ear specialist has made suggestions to the primary care physician regarding further management. When your child is being evaluated by an ear specialist, make sure the ear specialist stays in close contact with your child's primary care doctor. If a misunderstanding arises, request that the doctors communicate with each other and then inform you of their outcome.

Seeking a Second Opinion

A growing number of medical insurance companies are now requiring a second opinion before authorizing reimbursement for costs of a surgical procedure. Therefore, if a doctor wants to schedule your child for insertion of tubes in the ears, adenoidectomy or tonsillectomy, check the stipulations in your family medical insurance policy to see if a second opinion is required.

Even if your medical insurance company does not require it, you may want to seek a second opinion if you feel uneasy about your own or your child's interactions with a doctor. You and your child must have good rapport with any doctors who will be involved with care of your child's ear infections.

If you believe your child's ear problems need evaluation by an ear specialist, but your family physician or pediatrician is reluctant to refer your child to an ear specialist, ask your friends to give you the name of a good ear specialist and make an appointment to have your child evaluated.

If you do not like the personality of an ear specialist, ask your pediatrician or family physician to recommend another ear specialist.

The best way to know if you need a second opinion is to ask lots of questions. When the recommendations that have been made frighten you or do not make sense to you, you may want to get a second opinion. Many individuals believe that second opinions should be sought *whenever* surgery is recommended. Trust your own instincts! If you went to the trouble of reading this book, then you have acquired a fair amount of information about your child's ear infection. If it seems to you that a doctor is giving your child a cursory ear examination, if advice that you are receiving seems illogical, if you get the feeling that a doctor does not like answering your questions about reasons for a certain recommended treatment — you just might be right!

Never be embarrassed to seek a second opinion. Good doctors are not offended by a parent's desire to seek a second opinion. You have every right to ask all doctors who have been involved with care of your child to send pertinent records to the doctor who will be offering a second opinion. (Sometimes there may be a fee for preparation of medical records and summary letters that are sent by one doctor to another.) You can even ask one ear specialist to suggest the name of a colleague for a second opinion.

When the second opinion differs significantly from the first opinion, seek the help of your primary care physician in choosing the best approach to care for your child. When in doubt, trust your own instincts and go with the alternative that makes the most sense to you.

SUMMARY

You, as a parent, can play an important role in assuring that your child is receiving the best medical treatment possible. Remember these three important points:

Ask questions.   Make sure you understand the "who, what, why, when and how" of the condition and treatment. Don't be embarrassed to ask what you may think are "dumb" questions and don't think you are offending a physician by asking questions.

Don't be in a hurry.   In managing childhood ear infections, time is on your side. That is, you need not rush into a decision about prophylactic use of antibiotics or surgery. Make a decision only after seeking the advice of an ear specialist, after possibly seeking a second opinion, and after making sure you feel comfortable with the decision.

Trust your instincts.   If you have gone to the trouble of reading this book, then you have a very good fundamental understanding of childhood ear infections and can apply this information to your child's situation.

NOTES

1.   Cohn V. "Look, Doc, I've Been Meaning to Tell You . . ." The Washington Post Health Magazine. January 16, 1985.

2.   Bluestone CD. Otitis Media: Update 1984. Infectious Diseases. 1984 April: 14(4): 4.

3.   Bluestone CD, Klein JO. "Otitis Media with Effusion, Atelectasis and Eustachian Tube Dysfunction" in Pediatric Otolaryngology Volume 1 (edited by CD Bluestone and SE Stool). 1983 WB Saunders Co.: 434.

4.   Schwartz RH, Rodriguez WJ, Grundfast KM. Duration of middle ear effusion after acute otitis media. Pediatric Infectious Disease. 1984, Williams and Wilkins Co.:204–227.

5.   National Center for Health Statistics. Unpublished data from the National Ambulatory Medical Care Survey, 1980–81.

6.   David, CB; Hamrick, HJ; et al. "Follow-Up After Otitis Media." Letter to The New Eng J Med. 1982 July 22; 252.

7.   Shurin PA. "Inflammatory Diseases of the Nose and Paranasal Sinuses" in Pediatric Otolaryngology Vol. 1 (editors SA Stool and CD Bluestone). 1983: WB Saunders Co.: 781.

8.   Ginsburg, CM. Otitis Media. Pediatrics 1984;74 (suppl): 948–949.

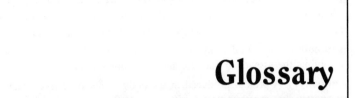

Glossary

Acoustic otoscope: An instrument that detects middle ear fluid by reflecting sound waves off the eardrum.

Acute: Severe and sharp, as in "acute" pain. Also, severe but of short duration, not chronic, such as "acute ear infection."

Acute otitis media: Rapid and immediate onset of signs and symptoms of infection in the middle ear that means infected fluid is pressing against the eardrum and causing ear pain.

Adenoids: Growths of lymphoid tissue in the upper part of the throat, behind the nose.

Adenoidectomy: Surgical removal of the adenoids.

Adhesive otitis media: Collapsed eardrum stuck to bones and membranes in the middle ear; can be an end-stage result of chronic inflammation and infection in the middle ear.

Aeration: In this book, the term refers to putting air back into the middle ear through forcible means (such as Politerization) or through surgical means (such as insertion of tympanostomy tubes).

Allergy: A hypersensitivity to a specific substance, such as pollen or mold, which in similar amounts is harmless to most people. As a result of the hypersensitivity, the person has a reaction such as sneezing, watery eyes or nasal congestion.

Amoxicillin: A penicillin that is the antibiotic most commonly prescribed by physicians in the treatment of otitis media.

Ampicillin: A penicillin used in the treatment of otitis media.

Analgesic (Greek: an—without; algesia—pain):   Pain reliever.

Anatomy: The science of the structure of animals and plants; the structure of an organism or body.

Anesthesia (Greek: an—without; aisthesis—feeling):   A loss of sensation induced by an anesthetic and limited to a specific area (local anesthesia) or involving a loss of consciousness (general anesthesia).

Antibiotic: A natural or synthetically-produced substance that destroys or inhibits the growth of bacteria and other microorganisms.

Antibody: A protein produced in the body in response to contact with an antigen that creates an immunity to the antigen.

Antihistamine: A drying agent for the nasal passages that blocks the effect of histamine.

Antigen: A substance, such as an enzyme or poison, to which the body reacts by producing an antibody.

Anvil: One of the three bones of the middle ear, also known as the incus.

Articulation: The process by which sounds, syllables and words are formed when your tongue, jaw, teeth, lips and palate alter the air stream coming from the vocal folds.

Aspirate: To remove by suction.

Atelectasis (Greek: a—without; telos—an end; aktasis—a stretching out):   The condition which describes the eardrum when it loses its thickness and tense quality and is sucked into the middle ear. Also known as a retracted eardrum.

Audiogram: A graph, made by an audiometer, showing the percentage of hearing loss in an ear.

Audiologist: A professional who specializes in the identification and prevention of hearing problems and in the non-medical rehabilitation of those who have a hearing impairment.

Audiometer: An instrument used to measure hearing through the use of controlled amounts of sound.

Auditory nerve: The nerve that emerges from the temporal bone and leads to the brain and which carries signals of sound to the brain; the eighth cranial nerve.

Augmentin®:   A new penicillin reportedly effective in treating otitis media, it contains clavulanic acid and is effective in killing bacteria resistant to penicillin.

Auricle (Latin: auris—ear): The external part of the ear, also called the pinna.

Bacampicillin®: A new penicillin reportedly effective in treating otitis media and supposedly effective in killing bacteria resistant to penicillin.

Bacteria: Microscopic organisms that can cause disease or are necessary for such functions as fermentation and nitrogen fixation.

Bactrim®: An antibiotic, used in the treatment of otitis media, that is made from a combination of trimethoprim and sulfamethoxazole.

Branhamella catarrhallis: A bacteria that causes otitis media.

Bottle propping: Lying a child on his back in bed and propping the bottle in his mouth for long periods of time.

Ceclor®: A cephalosporin antibiotic, used in the treatment of otitis media, whose generic name is cefaclor.

Cephalosporin: One family of antibiotic that includes Ceclor®.

Cerumen: Earwax; a yellowish, waxlike substance secreted by glands in the canal of the external ear.

Chemoprophylaxis: The prevention of a disease by the use of medication.

Cholesteatoma: An abnormal type of skin that gathers and starts to collect within the middle ear.

Cilia: Short, hairlike outgrowths of certain cells, capable of rhythmic beating that move fluids, such as mucus.

Cochlea (Greek: kochlias—snail): The spiral-shaped part of the inner ear, containing the auditory nerve endings.

Complication: A disease that occurs at the same time (concurrently with) another disease.

Conductive hearing loss: A type of hearing loss caused by limitation of vibration of the middle ear ossicles.

Corticosteroid: A medication, derived from the hormone prednisone, that helps to shrink swollen tissue. Scientists have been experimenting to find out whether this substance can be used to shrink swollen tissue in the eustachian tube.

Cps: The abbreviation for "cycles per second," this is a measurement for frequency of sound (the number of vibrations per unit of time).

Culture and sensitivity testing: A laboratory test in which a sample of middle ear fluid is tested to find out which antibiotic would be effective in killing bacteria found in the sample.

Curette:　A long, thin instrument with a tiny hook at the end used to clean out earwax from the external ear canal.

Cyclacillin®:　A new penicillin being tested for its effectiveness in treating otitis media.

dB:　The abbreviation for decibel, which is a unit in physics that measures sound pressure level.

Decongestant:　A medication that shrinks swollen mucous membranes and relieves nasal congestion.

Diagnosis:　The act or process of deciding the nature of a diseased condition by examination of the symptoms.

Down syndrome:　A congenital disease characterized by mental deficiency, a broad face and slanting eyes.

ENT specialist:　Abbreviation for ear, nose and throat specialist; an otolaryngologist.

Eardrum:　A broad, flat cone-shaped membrane that separates the outer ear canal from the middle ear; the tympanic membrane.

Ear Infection:　Inflammation of the middle ear caused by bacteria, virus or another microorganism.

Edema:　An abnormal accumulation of fluid in cells, tissues or cavities of the body, resulting in swelling.

Effusion:　The escape of fluid into a part of the body. Fluid in the middle ear is called middle ear effusion.

Eighth nerve (eighth cranial nerve):　The auditory nerve; it emerges from the temporal bone and leads to the brain, carrying signals of sound to the brain.

Erosion:　To deteriorate or decay, as in erosion (or dissolving) of the delicate middle ear bones.

Erythromycin:　One family of antibiotic that is combined with sulfisoxazole to make Pediazole®.

Eustachian tube:　A slender tube or canal with collapsible walls that links the middle ear with the nasopharynx.

External ear:　The auricle or pinna and the external ear canal.

Extrude:　Push or force out; expel; the process by which a tube emerges from the eardrum.

Frequency:　In physics, the number of vibrations per unit of time, measured in cycles per second (cps).

Frequently occurring otitis media: More than four ear infections in each of two consecutive seasons.

Gantrisin®: An antibiotic, used in the treatment of otitis media, made from acetyl sulfisoxazole. Often used for prophylactic treatment of frequently occurring acute otitis media.

Granulation: The formation of minute, rounded, fleshy tissue on the surface of inflamed tissue that is in the process of healing.

Grommet: A type of tube inserted into the eardrum to ventilate the middle ear; same as tympanostomy tube.

Hz: The abbreviation for Hertz; the international unit for frequency, equal to one cycle per second.

Hammer: One of the three bones of the middle ear, the malleus.

Hemophilus influenzae: One of the two types of bacteria that most commonly cause otitis media.

Histamine: A substance that causes congestion and which is released by body tissues during an allergic reaction.

Hyposensitization: To treat with frequent, small injections of an antigen so as to decrease the symptoms of an allergy to that antigen.

Immune response: The body's defense against illness that causes the body to recover from illness and protect against reinfection.

Immunity: Resistance or protection against a disease; power to resist infection, especially as a result of antibody formation.

Immunodeficiency: A condition that occurs when the immune system is not functioning properly.

Impedance audiometry: Measurement of the function of the middle ear and eardrum.

Incus: The central of the three small bones in the middle ear that is shaped somewhat like an anvil.

Indications: Criteria that "indicate" a surgery is needed.

Inflammation: A reaction to injury, infection or irritation by redness, pain, heat, swelling or loss of function.

Iontophoresis: A procedure that anesthesizes the eardrum by using an anesthetic liquid on the eardrum and then using electrical current to draw the anesthetic liquid through the eardrum.

Inner ear: That part of the ear responsible for hearing and balance that contains the cochlea, semicircular canals and the organ of Corti.

Intensity: In physics, the amount of sound per unit area.

Intermittent hearing loss: Hearing loss that comes and goes.

Labyrinthitis: Infection of the inner ear.

Language: A code that we learn to use in order to communicate ideas, such as reading, writing, gesturing and speaking.

Light reflex: The brilliant reflection of light directed onto the eardrum by an examining instrument.

Lumen: The opening of a hollow tube.

Lymphoid: Tissue of the lymph nodes which is any one of many small compact structures lying in groups along the course of the lymphatic vessels.

Mastoid: The portion of the temporal bone that forms the bony prominence that can be felt behind the ear.

Mastoiditis: Inflammation of the mastoid air cells, which are the spaces lined by mucous membrane in the mastoid bone.

Meningitis: An infection of the lining surrounding the brain, called the meninges.

Microbiology: The branch of biology that deals with microorganisms.

Microorganism or microbe: A microscopic animal or vegetable organism, such as bacteria, virus, or fungus.

Middle ear: Also called the tympanic cavity, this is a small air-filled chamber separated from the external ear by the eardrum. Extending across the chamber is a chain of three ossicles—the malleus, incus and stapes.

Middle ear ventilation disorder: A condition in which the eardrum is drawn into the middle ear space due to negative pressure; also called "retracted."

Mucoid: When used to describe the consistency of middle ear fluid, it means thick, viscid and mucus-like.

Mucolyctic agent: A substance that can reduce the thickness of mucus, and which has been found to be effective in thinning mucus. Some scientists are studying whether it can be effective in the treatment of otitis media.

Mucus: The thick, slimy secretion of the mucous membranes, that moistens and protects them.

Mucous membranes: A mucus-secreting membrane lining some body cavities and canals such as the nose, mouth and middle ear.

Myringotomy (Latin:myringa—eardrum; Greek:tome—excision): The surgical procedure performed by making a small incision in the eardrum with a surgical knife to allow the drainage of fluid.

Nasopharynx: The part of the pharynx lying directly behind the nasal passages and above the soft palate.

Negative pressure: A condition that develops when the air pressure outside the eardrum is greater than air pressure in the middle ear, causing the eardrum to be drawn in toward the middle ear cavity.

Occlude: To close, shut or block (a passage).

Organ of Corti: The receptive organ of hearing located within the cochlea of the inner ear.

Ossicles: The three tiniest bones in the body—the malleus, incus and stapes. In the middle ear, they form a bridge that connects the eardrum with the oval window.

Otalgia (Greek: oto—ear; algia—pain): pain in the ear, an earache.

Otitis externa (Greek: ot—ear; itis—inflammation; externa—exter nal): Inflammation of the outer ear, most often caused by water (often called swimmer's ear).

Otitis media (Greek: ot—ear; itis—inflammation; media—middle): Inflammation of the middle ear.

Otolaryngology (Greek: oto—ear; laryn—throat; logos-study); otorhinolaryngology (oto—ear; rhino—nose; laryn—throat; logos—study): The study of the ear, nose and throat.

Otolaryngologist: A specialist in disorders of the head and neck, especially those related to the ear, nose and throat.

Otorrhea (Greek: oto—ear; rhoia—flow): Discharge from the ear.

Otoscope: A magnifying instrument used to view the eardrum.

Oval window: An opening in the inner wall of the middle ear that communicates with the inner ear. The footplate of the stapes fits into the oval window.

P.E. tube: "Pressure equalization" tube, same as tympanostomy tube.

Palate: The roof of the mouth.

Patent (pronounced like "latent"): Open.

Pathogen: Any microorganism or virus that can cause disease.

Pediazole®: An antibiotic, made of a combination of erythromycin and sulfisoxazole, used in the treatment of otitis media.

Penicillin: One family of antibiotic that includes amoxicillin.

Perforation: When used in reference to the eardrum, it means a hole in the eardrum.

Permeable: Open to passage or penetration.

Persistent middle ear fluid: The presence of fluid in one or both ears for more than 10 weeks.

Physiology: The branch of biology dealing with the functions and vital processes of living organisms or their parts and organs.

Pinna: The external ear, also known as the auricle.

Pitch: The quality of tone or sound determined by the frequency of vibration of the sound waves reaching the ear; the greater the frequency, the higher the pitch.

Pneumatic otoscope: Attached to this otoscope is a tube or a rubber bulb through which the physician can gently blow or squeeze air into the ear canal to test movement of the eardrum.

Politzerization: A method of inflating the middle ear in which an aspirator is used to squeeze air through the nose while the person swallows.

Primary care physician: A personal physician. Pediatricians and family physicians are primary care physicians who provide medical care for children.

Prophylaxis: The prevention of a disease with the use of medication.

Purulent: When used to describe the consistency of middle ear fluid, it means puslike.

Resistant: In this book, the term is used in relation to bacteria that can remain alive in the presence of an antibiotic.

Retracted eardrum: An eardrum which is drawn into the middle ear chamber.

Round window: An opening in the inner wall of the middle ear that communicates with the inner ear. The round window is beneath the oval window and is closed over by a small fibrous disc called the secondary drum membrane.

Sensorineural hearing loss: A hearing loss that occurs when the inner ear is damaged.

Septra®: An antibiotic, used in the treatment of otitis media, that is made from a combination of trimethoprim and sulfamethoxazole.

Sequelea: An unwanted condition, illness or disease that follows and is caused by another disease process.

Serous: When used to describe the consistency of middle ear fluid, it means thin and watery.

Side effects: A term used to describe adverse effects, such as diarrhea or skin rashes, that occur in reaction to antibiotics.

Speculum: A hollow funnel-shaped instrument through which a doctor can view the eardrum.

Speech: The spoken form of language.

Speech-language pathologist: A specialist trained to identify problem areas in speech and language and to determine the direction for therapy to correct the problems.

Stapes: The innermost of a chain of three bones in the middle ear shaped like a stirrup.

Stirrup: Same as stapes.

Streptococcus pneumoniae: One of the two most common bacteria found to cause otitis media.

Sulfonamides: The so-called sulfa drugs; includes Bactrim®, Septra® and Gantrisin®.

Suppurative: A word often used in describing otitis media, meaning "forming pus." Some physicians use it in describing acute otitis media.

Susceptible: In this book, the term is used to describe bacteria killed by an antibiotic.

Symptom: A condition that accompanies a disease and which indicates the disease's presence—an earache is a symptom of an ear infection.

Temporal bone: The cavities of the middle and inner ear are contained in this bone, which forms part of the side wall as well as the base of the skull.

Tonsils: A pair of oval masses of lymphoid tissue, one on each side of the throat at the back of the mouth.

Tonsillectomy: Removal of the tonsils.

Toynbee maneuver: A method to forcibly inflate the middle ear by swallowing while the nostrils are closed and swallowing simultaneously while blowing against the closed nostrils.

Tube: Same as tympanostomy tube.

Tuning fork: A small steel instrument with two prongs, which when struck sounds a certain fixed tone in perfect pitch; used to estimate hearing ability in older children.

Tympanic membrane (Greek: tympanal—drum): Commonly called the eardrum, it is a broad, flat, cone-shaped membrane that separates the outer ear canal from the middle ear.

Tympanocentesis: The procedure by which a physician aspirates middle ear fluid through an opening made with a needle in the eardrum.

Tympanogram: A curve, charted on a piece of paper by a tympanometer, which shows the movement of the middle ear system.

Tympanometer: An instrument used to measure the physical properties of the middle ear and eardrum.

Tympanosclerosis: Chalky white plaques or deposits on the eardrum or in the middle ear.

Tympanostomy tube: A tiny tube surgically implanted in the ear drum to provide ventilation for the middle ear.

Upper respiratory infection: The common cold.

Vaccine: An injection of a serum that artifically creates the immune response in the body to fight a specific disease.

Ventilation tube: Same as tympanostomy tube.

Virus: A group of microorganisms that cause disease in animals, such as measles, mumps or the common cold.

White blood cells: These components of the blood leave the blood stream and gather in large numbers in an infected area, where they aid in overcoming infection.

Index

Warner Shows You How to be a Successful Parent

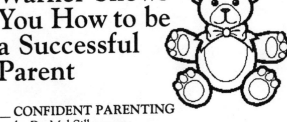

__ **CONFIDENT PARENTING**
by Dr. Mel Silberman
(U38-670, $5.95, U.S.A.) (U38-671, $8.95, Canada)

A family therapist speaks plainly to parents on how to be an effective and confident parent.

__ **JOAN LUNDEN'S MOTHER'S MINUTES**
by Michael Krauss and Joan Lunden with Sue Castle
(U38-257, $8.95, U.S.A.) (U38-258, $11.95, Canada)

A childcare book with sound, practical advice for safe, effective and happy parenting by one of television's most notable working mothers.

__ **THE NURTURING FATHER**
by Kyle D. Pruett, M.D.
(U38-662, $9.95, U.S.A.) (U38-663, $13.50, Canada)

A significant study that reveals the amazing effects on fathers, mothers, babies and society when male parents stay home to care for their children.

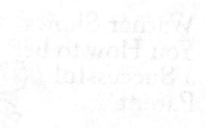

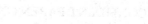